Multiple Choice Questions in Veterinary Nursing

Volume 2

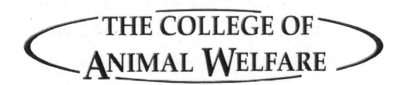

Multiple Choice Questions in Veterinary Nursing

Volume 2

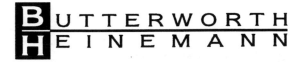

Butterworth-Heinemann
Linacre House, Jordan Hill, Oxford OX2 8DP
A division of Reed Educational and Professional Publishing Ltd

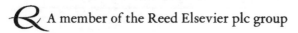 A member of the Reed Elsevier plc group

OXFORD BOSTON JOHANNESBURG
MELBOURNE NEW DELHI SINGAPORE

First published 1997

©College of Animal Welfare 1997

British Library Cataloguing in Publication Data
A catalogue record for this book is available from the British Library

Library of Congress Cataloguing in Publication Data
A catalogue record for this book is available from the Library of Congress

ISBN 0 7506 3612 2

Typeset by Mike Pearson c/o The College of Animal Welfare
Printed and bound in Great Britain by Biddles Ltd., Guildford and Kings Lynn

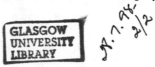

Contents

Acknowledgements

The college is most grateful for the help of the following colleagues in the preparation of this book.

A.J. Pearson BA VetMB MRCVS
College of Animal Welfare

B. Cooper VN Cert Ed
College of Animal Welfare

B. Drysdale VN Cert Ed
College of Animal Welfare

A. Jeffery VN Dip AVN (Surg)
College of Animal Welfare

B.J. White VN Cert Ed
College of Animal Welfare

Preface

The Part II examination was first introduced in January 1993 necessitating a book of multiple choice questions focusing on the Veterinary Nurse syllabus. You will find a complete list of the syllabus areas covered by the book in the table of contents.

Format of the Multiple Choice Examinations

The Royal College of Veterinary Surgeons Part 2 Veterinary Nurse multiple choice examination consists of two papers:

Paper I Medical Nursing, Diagnostic Aids & Radiography
Paper II Surgical, Obstetrical & Paediatric Nursing

Each paper contains 90 multiple choice questions which should be completed within a 90 minute period.

Recommended texts

Lane & Cooper (1994)
Veterinary Nursing, 6th edition
Butterworth-Heinemann, Oxford

Simpson G. (1994)
Practical Veterinary Nursing, 3rd edition
British Small Animal Veterinary Association, Cheltenham

Bishop, Y. (1996)
The Veterinary Formulary, 3rd edition
Pharmaceutical Press, London

Cochran, P.E. (1991)
Guide to Veterinary Medical Terminology
American Veterinary Publications, Goleta

Introduction

How the book is organised

This book of multiple choice questions for Part 2 student veterinary nurses has been produced in response to many, many requests.

It contains 350 questions, divided into subject sections. After the questions are firstly a list of correct answers, and then answers with comments and explanations — though not for all of them.

How to use the book

Do your revision first, then select 90 question numbers at random from the appropriate sections. Do this without looking at the questions in advance. You should be able to finish a 90 question test in 90 minutes. Once you have marked the paper, check the answers with comments for any further explanations you may need.

Questions

General Nursing

1) A 15 kg dog requires Pethidine at 2 mg/kg. The pethidine is supplied as a 50 mg/ml solution. How much is required?

   a) 0.3 ml
   b) 0.6 ml
   c) 1.0 ml
   d) 1.6 ml.

2) A 2.5% solution contains

   a) 2.5 g of solute in 1000 ml solvent
   b) 2.5 g of solute in 100 ml solvent
   c) 25 mg of solute in 1000 ml solvent
   d) 25 mg of solute in 100 ml solvent.

3) A 30 kg dog requires injections three times daily at a dose rate of 25 mg/kg/24 hours. The drug is in a 5% solution. What volume should be given each time?

   a) 2 ml
   b) 3 ml
   c) 4 ml
   d) 5 ml.

4)   A 40 kg dog requires injections two times daily at a drug
        dose rate of 25 mg/kg/24 hours. The drug is a suspension
        containing 150 mg/ml. What volume should be given each
        time?
        a) 2.5 ml
        b) 3.3 ml
        c) 4.0 ml
        d) 5 ml.

5)   A cat weighs 4.0 kg, and needs an antibiotic by mouth at
        50 mg/kg/24 hours for 10 days — to be divided to give two
        daily doses. The tablets available are 100 mg. How many
        tablets will be required for the course?
        a) 10
        b) 20
        c) 30
        d) 40.

6)   Epistaxis is
        a) an inability to stand up
        b) bleeding from the ears
        c) bleeding from the nostrils
        d) persistent vomiting.

7)   Following urinary catheterisation, systemic antibiotics
        should be given
        a) if the catheter is indwelling
        b) if blood is seen in the urine or on the catheter
        c) should the animal require repeated catheterisations
        d) in every case.

8)   For injection, you are given a drug in a 7.5% solution. The
        dose required for the dog you are treating is 10 mg/kg and
        the dog weighs 18 kg. What volume of the drug should you
        give?
        a) 1.2 ml
        b) 2.4 ml
        c) 3.6 ml
        d) 4.8 ml.

9) How much Dextrose powder is required to make up 50 ml of a 2.5% solution?
    a) 1.25 g
    b) 2.5 g
    c) 12.5 g
    d) 25 g.

10) How much of a drug would you give to an animal weighing 20 kg if the dose rate was 50 mg/kg and was presented as a 10% solution?
    a) 2.5 ml
    b) 10 ml
    c) 15 ml
    d) 20 ml.

11) Hydropropulsion is
    a) swimming physiotherapy
    b) the use of water as an aerosol, as in ultrasonic dental scalers
    c) using a stream of water, introduced into a urinary catheter, to try to force a urethral obstruction (e.g. a urinary calculus) back into the bladder
    d) using cold water to cool an animal with hyperthermia.

12) To which class of drugs does frusemide belong?
    a) Corticosteroids
    b) Diuretics
    c) Narcotic analgesics
    d) NSAIDS.

13) Which ONE of the following enteral feeding tubes does NOT normally require a general anaesthetic for its placement?
    a) Duodostomy tube
    b) Gastrostomy tube
    c) Nasogastric tube
    d) Pharyngostomy tube.

3

14) Which ONE of the following is a common indicator of pain in small animals?
   a) Bradycardia
   b) Brick red mucous membranes
   c) Pupillary constriction
   d) Tachypnoea.

15) Which ONE of the following methods of providing enteral nutrition carries with it the risk of peritonitis?
   a) Gastrostomy tube
   b) Nasogastric tube
   c) Orogastric tube
   d) Pharyngostomy tube.

16) Which ONE of the following might be part of the after-care for a patient following anal sac surgery?
   a) Enema
   b) Faecal consistency regulator
   c) Kaolin mixture
   d) Purgative.

17) Which ONE of the following statements concerning ill and recumbent animals is the LEAST accurate?
   a) Recumbent animals have a reduced requirement for calories, as they are expending little energy
   b) Ill and recumbent animals often require increased protein in the diet, to cope with tissue breakdown and repair
   c) Ill and recumbent animals require reduced amounts of protein in the diet
   d) Ill and recumbent animals should have reduced carbohydrate in the diet to avoid obesity.

18) Which ONE of the following statements is the MOST accurate, concerning the nursing of a recumbent dog?

   a) Long term recumbent patients should not be paid an excessive amount of attention, as they do not learn then to settle quietly in their kennel

   b) Recumbent animals take up less nursing time than an active post-operative patient

   c) The dog should be positioned in a quiet area, where it is not over-stimulated by constant activity outside its kennel

   d) The dog will often appreciate being housed where it can see a lot of activity going on, and passing people can talk to it. This helps relieve boredom.

19) Which of the following is NOT a good choice as an enema solution in a very young cat?

   a) Mineral oil

   b) Liquid paraffin

   c) Saline solution

   d) Warm water.

20) Which of the following is the LEAST valuable in the prevention and treatment of decubitus ulcers in the recumbent patient?

   a) Deep, soft bedding

   b) Harden any areas of skin which look likely to develop ulcers by the regular application of surgical spirit

   c) Protection on bony prominences with padded dressings

   d) Regular massage of areas at risk.

21) Which of the following is not important in the prevention of hypostatic pneumonia in a recumbent animal?

   a) Encourage the animal to lie in sternal rather than lateral recumbency

   b) Carry out daily effluage

   c) Stimulate coughing by daily coupage

   d) Turn the animal at least every four hours.

22) *Coupage* is
  a) the debriding of a contaminated wound and the removal of devitalised tissue before suturing
  b) the flushing of a contaminated wound to remove particulate debris
  c) the placement of a surgical drain
  d) vigorously hitting the chest with cupped hand in order to to stimulate the circulation, and reduce the pooling of blood in the lungs of an inactive animal.

Fluid Therapy

23) A dehydrated 10 kg dog is placed on an intravenous drip at 1.5 times maintenance. What is the total daily volume required, and what should the drip rate be, if the giving set delivers 15 drops per ml?
  a) 300 ml total, at approximately 6 drops per minute
  b) 300 ml total, at approximately 12 drops per minute
  c) 600 ml total, at approximately 6 drops per minute
  d) 600 ml total, at approximately 12 drops per minute.

24) At what percentage dehydration does loss of skin elasticity first occur in a dehydrated animal?
  a) 2%
  b) 5%
  c) 7%
  d) 10%.

Warning: illegal if copied

25) Following a road traffic accident, a dog is put on a drip, and a manometer is set up to measure CVP. After a while, the CVP is measured, and is found to be 2 cm water. Which ONE of the following is the CORRECT conclusion from this observation?

   a) The animal is suffering from congestive heart failure
   b) The blood pressure is now normal, so fluid administration can be stopped
   c) The dog is in danger of over-hydration. Renal function should be checked
   d) The dog is still suffering from reduced blood volume, and more fluids should be administered.

26) How much 50% dextrose solution must be added to a bag of sterile water (once an identical volume of water has been withdrawn) to make 500 ml of a 2.5% dextrose solution?

   a) 12.5 ml
   b) 25 ml
   c) 50 ml
   d) 100 ml.

27) In the assessment of the degree of fluid deficit, tenting skin, and a capillary refill time of more than 2 seconds suggests a deficit of approximately

   a) 5%
   b) 5–8%
   c) 10–12%
   d) 12–15%.

28) Plasma may be stored at

   a) -70 deg C for 6 months before use
   b) +4 deg C for 6 weeks before use
   c) +4 deg C for 3 weeks before use
   d) at room temperature for up to 24 hours before use.

29) The largest fluid compartment in the body is the
   a) extracellular fluid
   b) interstitial fluid
   c) intracellular fluid
   d) plasma water.

30) What is the maximum number of days that an intravenous catheter should be left in place?
   a) 2
   b) 4
   c) 6
   d) 8.

31) What is the normal pH of plasma in the dog?
   a) 7.2–7.25
   b) 7.25–7.3
   c) 7.3–7.35
   d) 7.35–7.4.

32) What is the normal range of central venous pressure in a healthy dog?
   a) 3–7 mm water
   b) 3–7 mm mercury
   c) 3–7 cm water
   d) 3–7 cm mercury.

33) Which ONE of the following anticoagulants is normally used for collecting blood for transfusion?
   a) Citrate
   b) EDTA
   c) Fluoride
   d) Heparin.

34) Which ONE of the following conditions is MOST likely to lead to metabolic alkalosis?
   a) Apnoea
   b) Diarrhoea
   c) Hypoglycaemia
   d) Vomiting.

35) Which ONE of the following is a crystalloid solution?
   a) Dextran
   b) Haemaccel
   c) 0.9% Sodium chloride
   d) Whole blood.

36) Which ONE of the following is hypertonic with respect to plasma?
   a) Dextran 70
   b) Haemaccel
   c) 0.18% NaCl with 4% Dextrose
   d) 0.9% NaCl.

37) Which ONE of the following is the main cation in intracellular fluid?
   a) Calcium
   b) Magnesium
   c) Potassium
   d) Sodium.

38) Which ONE of the following is the route of inevitable fluid loss?
   a) In vomitus
   b) The gastro-intestinal tract
   c) The respiratory tract
   d) The urinary tract.

39) Which ONE of the following pairs of ions are MOST abundant in plasma?
   a) Potassium and chloride
   b) Potassium and phosphate
   c) Sodium and bicarbonate
   d) Sodium and chloride.

40) Which ONE of the following statements about a burette giving set is the MOST accurate?
   a) Fluids can be given very rapidly
   b) It should always be used when giving a blood transfusion
   c) Small volumes can be given accurately
   d) The apparatus can be set to heat the fluid before it reaches the
   patient.

41) Which ONE of the following fluids is MOST suitable for use
subcutaneously in a rabbit or guinea pig?
   a) 5% Dextrose
   b) Hartmann's solution
   c) 0.18% NaCl with 4% dextrose
   d) Any of the above.

42) Which ONE of the following fluids is the MOST suitable for
use in a case of dehydration following severe diarrhoea?
   a) 0.9% NaCl
   b) Hartmann's solution
   c) 0.18% NaCl + 4% Dextrose
   d) Ringer's solution.

43) Which of the following statements is the LEAST accurate?
   a) PCV can be used to estimate fluid deficit, but will not be accurate in animals suffering from anaemia
   b) PCV can give an accurate measure of fluid deficit as it rises by
   1% for each 10 ml/kg fluid loss
   c) PCV can only be used to give a rough estimate of fluid deficit,
   as the normal PCV varies from individual to individual
   d) PCV is of most use in assessing the degree of dehydration if the
   individual's normal PCV is known.

44) Which ONE of the following is the MOST LIKELY risk during or after intra-osseous fluid administration?
   a) Acidosis
   b) Infection
   c) Local irritation
   d) Overhydration.

45) Which of the following is NEVER a sign of an incompatibility reaction after a blood transfusion?

   a) diarrhoea
   b) haemoglobinuria
   c) tachycardia
   d) vomiting.

Diagnostic Aids

46) A laboratory test shows an increase in serum protein. Which ONE of the following is a possible cause?

   a) Anaemia
   b) Dehydration
   c) Over-hydration
   d) Renal failure.

47) How long can a serum sample be stored in a refrigerator without deterioration?

   a) A few hours only
   b) 3 days
   c) 7 days
   d) 28 days.

48) Howell Jolly bodies are

   a) nuclear remnants in young erythrocytes
   b) signs of intracellular parasites of red cells
   c) small sections of neutrophil segmented nuclei
   d) erythrocytes of a cheerful disposition.

49) Into which anticoagulant would you collect dog or cat blood for routine haematological examination?

   a) EDTA
   b) Heparin
   c) Sodium citrate
   d) Sodium fluoride.

50) Leishman's stain is commonly used for
   a) bacterial stain
   b) differential white cell count
   c) identifying red blood cells
   d) urinalysis.

51) Polycythaemia is
   a) an increase in the number of platelets
   b) an increase in the number of red blood cells
   c) an increase in the number of white blood cells
   d) variable sizes of red blood cells in the blood.

52) Routine haematological examination reveals the following: low PCV, low rbc, relatively high reticulocyte count. Which ONE of the following is the MOST likely cause of the animal's condition?
   a) Bone marrow hypoplasia
   b) Chronic renal disease
   c) FeLV
   d) Road traffic accident.

53) Specimens for toxicological examination should be preserved in
   a) ethanol
   b) formal saline
   c) formalin
   d) neutral buffered formalin.

54) Sudan III is used in the laboratory to estimate the quantity of which ONE of the following?
   a) Faecal fat
   b) Protein in urine
   c) Reticulocytes in peripheral blood
   d) Serum bicarbonate.

55) The maximum volume of fluid that should be contained in a *pathological specimen* container to be sent through the post is
    a) 20 ml
    b) 50 ml
    c) 100 ml
    d) 200 ml.

56) What does ELISA stand for?
    a) Enzyme-leukaemia immune assay
    b) Enzyme-leukaemia immunosorbent assay
    c) Enzyme-linked immune assay
    d) Enzyme-linked immunosorbent assay.

57) What does the term *Rouleaux* mean?
    a) A stain used to detect blood parasites
    b) Grouping of red blood cells in stacks
    c) Nuclear remnants in a cell
    d) Red blood cells showing irregular margins and prickly edges.

58) What is the correct method for the disposal of culture plates?
    a) Autoclave and put in a black bag
    b) Autoclave and put in a clinical waste bag
    c) Disinfect and put in a clinical waste bag
    d) In a clinical waste bag.

59) What is the normal range for packed cell volume in the dog?
    a) 25–45%
    b) 37–55%
    c) 40–58%
    d) 45–62%.

60) Which ONE of the following may cause haemolysis in a blood sample?
    a) Leaving the plasma unseparated in transit
    b) The use of too fine a needle
    c) Water on the needle or syringe
    d) All of the above.

61) Which ONE of the following media would you use to isolate fungi?
   a) Chocolate agar
   b) Deoxycholate-citrate agar
   c) MacConkey's broth
   d) Sabouraud's agar.

62) Which ONE of the following preservatives is best for a urine sample to be sent for bacteriological examination?
   a) Boric acid
   b) Formalin
   c) Thymol
   d) Toluene.

63) Which ONE of the following statements is NOT true?
   a) Eosinophilia is often found in cases of parasitism
   b) Lymphopaenia may be found in chemotherapy patients
   c) Neutropaenia is usually seen in infectious inflammatory conditions
   d) Thrombocytopaenia may result in haemorrhage.

64) Which of the following blood parameters would you expect to increase significantly following a road traffic accident resulting in a fractured femur and significant muscle damage?
   a) ALT
   b) Cholesterol
   c) CK
   d) SAP.

65) Which ONE of the following conditions is likely to lead to an increase in BUN?
   a) High protein, low-carbohydrate diet
   b) Renal failure
   c) Urethral obstruction
   d) All of the above.

66)   Which ONE of the following media would you use to isolate salmonella?

a) Blood agar
b) MacConkey's broth
c) Nutrient agar
d) Selenite broth.

67)   Which reagents are necessary for performing a Gram's stain?

a) Carbol fuschin, acid alcohol, methylene blue
b) Carbol fuschin, Lugol's iodine, methylene blue and acetone
c) Crystal violet, Lugol's iodine, acetone and saffranine
d) Crystal violet, methylene blue, acetone and saffranine.

Medical Nursing

Parasitology

68)   A fluid filled cyst containing a single invaginated tapeworm scolex attached to the cyst wall is called a

a) coenurus
b) cysticercoid
c) cysticercus
d) hydatid.

69)   *Aelurostrongylus abstrusus* is

a) diagnosed by the presence of larvae in the faeces of the cat
b) not found in the United Kingdom
c) the cause of heartworm in dogs
d) the common bladder worm of the dog, the eggs being passed in the urine of an affected dog.

70)   All classes of insecticides may affect the CNS except

a) carbamates
b) insect growth regulators
c) organophosphates
d) pyrethrins.

71)   *Dipylidium caninum* infestation causes disease in the final host by
        a) causing diarrhoea
        b) competition for nutrients with the host
        c) loss of blood from the intestinal wall
        d) *Dipylidium caninum* rarely causes overt disease in the final host.

72)   Name two cestodes that may be found in the dog and cat.
        a) *Dipylidium caninum* and *Taenia taeniaeformis*
        b) *Dipylidium caninum* and *Trichuris vulpis*
        c) *Trichuris vulpis* and *Toxocara canis*
        d) *Uncinaria stenocephala* and *Taenia taeniaeformis*.

73)   Pups may have adult worms of *Toxocara canis* within their intestines by the time they are how old?
        a) Ten days
        b) Three weeks
        c) Five weeks
        d) Eight weeks.

74)   The active ingredient in *Droncit* is
        a) fenbendazole
        b) mebendazole
        c) nitroscanate
        d) praziquantel.

75)   The active ingredient in *Nuvan Top* is
        a) dichlorvos
        b) methoprene
        c) permethrin
        d) pybuthrin.

76)   The active ingredient in *Panacur* is
        a) fenbendazole
        b) mebendazole
        c) nitroscanate
        d) oxfendazole.

Warning: illegal if copied

77) The flea species found MOST commonly on pet dogs is
   a) *Aracheopsyllus erinachiae*
   b) *Ctenocephalides canis*
   c) *Ctenocephalides felis*
   d) *Pulex irritans.*

78) The infective stage of the *Toxocara canis* larva is
   a) L1
   b) L2
   c) L3
   d) L4.

79) The intermediate host of *Taenia ovis* is the
   a) cow
   b) rabbit
   c) rat or mouse
   d) sheep.

80) The intermediate host of *Taenia pisiformis* is the
   a) cow
   b) rabbit
   c) rat or mouse
   d) sheep.

81) The intermediate host of *Taenia serialis* is
   a) cow
   b) rabbit
   c) rat or mouse
   d) sheep.

82) The larvae of *Toxocara canis* pass from the bitch to the intra-uterine pups from approximately which day of pregnancy onwards?
   a) 32 days
   b) 37 days
   c) 42 days
   d) 47 days.

83) Each individual tapeworm segment is called a
    a) coenurus
    b) proglottid
    c) rostellum
    d) scolex.

84) The scientific name for the cat lungworm is
    a) *Aelurostrongylus abstrusus*
    b) *Angiostrongylus vasorum*
    c) *Filaroides osleri*
    d) *Oslerus osleri.*

85) The scientific name for the dog whipworm is
    a) *Ancylostoma caninum*
    b) *Dirofilaria immitis*
    c) *Trichuris vulpis*
    d) *Uncinaria stenocephala.*

86) The *Taenia* species that MOST commonly has the cat as its final host is
    a) *hydatigena*
    b) *ovis*
    c) *serialis*
    d) *taeniaeformis.*

87) What type of light is produced by a Wood's lamp?
    a) Infra-red
    b) Infra-red and ultra-violet
    c) Ultra-violet
    d) Ultra-violet and visible light.

88) Which ONE of the following drugs is NOT effective against cestodes?
    a) Fenbendazole
    b) Niclosamide
    c) Praziquantel
    d) Pyrental.

89) Which ONE of the following drugs is NOT effective against nematodes?
   a) Mebendazole
   b) Oxfendazole
   c) Piperazine
   d) Praziquantel.

90) Which ONE of the following is NOT a route of infection of *Toxocara cati* in a kitten?
   a) Ingestion of a paratenic host
   b) Ingestion of L2 larva from the environment
   c) Intra-uterine infection
   d) Trans-mammary infection.

91) Which ONE of the following is NOT a surface living mite?
   a) *Cheyletiella*
   b) *Cnemidocoptes*
   c) *Otodectes*
   d) *Trombicula autumnalis.*

92) Which ONE of the following is a sensible precaution for a pregnant woman to take to avoid infection with *Toxoplasma gondii*?
   a) Avoid eating sheep cheeses
   b) Have the family's cats blood tested for Toxoplasmosis
   c) Wear rubber gloves when gardening
   d) All of the above.

93) *Uncinaria stenocephala* is most likely to cause
   a) elephantiasis in dogs from West Africa
   b) heartworm
   c) pedal dermatitis in kennelled dogs
   d) severe diarrhoea.

94) Which ONE of the following is not an ascarid worm?
   a) *Capillaria plica*
   b) *Toxascaris leonina*
   c) *Toxocara canis*
   d) *Toxocara cati.*

19

95)   Which ONE of the following parasites can NOT be diagnosed by a skin scraping or brushing?
   a) *Cheyletiella*
   b) *Dipylidium caninum*
   c) *Helminth dermatoses*
   d) *Sarcoptes scabiei.*

96)   Which ONE of the following parasites is NOT found in Great Britain?
   a) *Ancylostoma caninum*
   b) *Dirofilaria immitis*
   c) *Trichuris vulpis*
   d) *Uncinaria stenocephala.*

97)   Which ONE of the following parasites is found living within hair follicles?
   a) *Cnemidocoptes*
   b) *Demodex*
   c) *Notoedres*
   d) *Sarcoptes.*

98)   Which ONE of the following statements about Hydatid disease is NOT true?
   a) Man can be the final host of the parasite
   b) The adult tapeworm is less than 1 cm long
   c) The sheep is the intermediate host of the parasite
   d) Within the United Kingdom, the parasite is found mainly in Wales and the west of the United Kingdom.

99)   Which ONE of the following statements about *Toxocara canis* is NOT true?
   a) After about eight weeks of age, most of the ingested larvae pass directly from the intestine to muscle, where they encyst
   b) In ideal conditions, a fertile *Toxocara canis* egg may develop to the infective stage in less than a week
   c) Puppies begin to develop immunity to *T. canis* from about seven weeks of age
   d) *Toxocara eggs* remain viable within the environment for up to two years.

100) Which ONE of the following statements about *Toxoplasma gondii* is NOT true?
   a) Boiling water is effective in killing *T. gondii* oocysts
   b) *T. gondii* is a common cause of abortion in sheep
   c) The final host of *T.gondii* is the cat
   d) To avoid infection, women are advised to avoid eating red meat during pregnancy.

101) Which ONE of the following statements about *Toxoplasma gondii* is the LEAST accurate?
   a) Asexual reproduction occurs in the tissues of intermediate hosts
   b) Infection is possible from one intermediate host to another, without the parasite passing through the final host
   c) Oocysts passed in the faeces take at least three weeks to become infective
   d) Sexual reproduction occurs only in the cat.

102) Which ONE of the following statements about cat lungworm infection is the LEAST accurate?
   a) Fenbendazole is effective against cat lungworm
   b) Infection with only a few worms will cause severe coughing
   c) Lungworm is probably under-diagnosed in the UK, with probably many more cats affected than is realised
   d) The adult worm produces larvae rather than eggs, which are coughed up and then swallowed by the cat.

103) Which ONE of the following statements about the use of Grisovin is NOT true?
   a) A long course of Grisovin (c. one month) is usually needed to clear a case of ringworm
   b) Grisovin may be teratogenic
   c) Grisovin may be used topically or parenterally
   d) Grisovin may cause enteric disturbances.

21

104) Which ONE of the following statements concerning *Echinococcus granulosus* is NOT true?
   a) Even a few worms in the final host can cause severe diarrhoea
   b) Only one of the two sub-species of *E.granulosus* is thought to be zoonotic
   c) The adult worm is about 0.5 cm long
   d) Within Britain, hydatid disease is most common in Wales.

105) Which ONE of the following statements is NOT true?
   a) Adult ticks have four pairs of legs
   b) All mites that affect cats are permanent parasites
   c) Juvenile ticks have only three pairs of legs
   d) Only the immature form of *Trombicula autumnalis* is parasitic.

106) Which ONE of the following statements is the most accurate?
   a) *Dipylidium caninum* may affect humans
   b) *Dipylidium caninum* may affect the cat as well as the dog
   c) The louse may be an intermediate host of *Dipylidium caninum*
   d) All of the above.

107) Whipworms are mainly found
   a) in kennelled dogs kept on concrete
   b) in kennelled dogs with access to permanent grass runs
   c) in dogs that have access to sheep carcasses
   d) in Wales.

Infectious Diseases

108) *Dermatophytosis* is the correct term for
   a) contact dermatitis
   b) food hypersensitivity affecting the skin
   c) fungal skin infection
   d) generalised pyoderma.

109) A dog belonging to a family is diagnosed as having lep-
tospirosis. Which ONE of the following pieces of ad-
vice/information should you give the family?
   a) Having had the disease, the dog will be solidly immune, so will
       no longer require annual vaccination against this disease
   b) The disease is a zoonosis, so they should all seek medical advice
   c) There is no further risk of infection once the dog is clinically
       recovered, as it will no longer be excreting the organism
   d) All of the above.

110) A suitable disinfectant for cleaning parvovirus-contaminated
areas is
   a) cetrimide
   b) chlorhexidine
   c) hypochlorite
   d) pine oil disinfectants.

111) Bacteria that are spherical in shape and arranged in groups
are known as
   a) bacilli
   b) spirochaetes
   c) staphylococci
   d) streptococci.

112) Canine parvovirus is closely related to
   a) feline infectious anaemia
   b) feline infectious enteritis
   c) rinderpest
   d) measles.

113) Canine parvovirus was first seen in the UK in
   a) 1974
   b) 1978
   c) 1982
   d) 1986.

114) Cats suffering from chlamydiosis generally
   a) are very listless and dull
   b) have a purulent conjunctivitis
   c) have diarrhoea
   d) all of the above.

115) Cerebellar hypoplasia in kittens may be caused by infection while *in utero* by
   a) FeLV
   b) FCV
   c) FIA
   d) FIE.

116) Endotoxins are
   a) poisonous substances produced within bacteria and liberated when the bacterium dies
   b) poisonous substances secreted by living bacterial cells
   c) substances produced by the body (or manufactured synthetically) to counteract the toxins produced by bacteria
   d) none of the above.

117) Feline infectious peritonitis is caused by
   a) a coronavirus
   b) a lentivirus
   c) a retrovirus
   d) an oncornavirus.

118) Feline leukaemia is caused by
   a) a calicivirus
   b) a coronavirus
   c) a lentivirus
   d) a retrovirus.

119) Feline infectious peritonitis is particularly common in
   a) Burmese cats
   b) Maine Coon cats
   c) Persian cats
   d) Siamese cats.

120) For which ONE of the following respiratory-disease causing organisms is no vaccine currently available?
   a) *Bordatella bronchiseptica*
   b) Canine adenovirus
   c) Canine herpesvirus
   d) Canine parainfluenza virus.

121) Infectious canine hepatitis has an incubation period of approximately
   a) 2–3 days
   b) 5–9 days
   c) 10–14 days
   d) 14–21 days.

122) Most cases of canine distemper are seen in dogs between the ages of 3 and 9 months old. This is because
   a) immunity to distemper takes a long time to become established following vaccination
   b) maternal immunity to distemper often persists for several months, so interfering with the development of active immunity following vaccination
   c) the dogs that catch distemper have usually lost their maternal immunity and have not been vaccinated, and are too young for immunity to field virus to have become established
   d) young dogs are still likely to have high levels of roundworm which debilitate them.

123) Most outbreaks of canine distemper in this country occur
   a) in boarding kennels
   b) in breeding kennels
   c) in rural areas
   d) in urban areas.

124) Rabies is now being controlled in much of Europe by
   a) killing the majority of foxes, which are the main reservoir of the disease
   b) vaccination of all domestic pets against the disease
   c) vaccination of foxes using an oral vaccine
   d) all of the above.

125) Rubarth's disease is
   a) an early term for FIA
   b) an inherited blood clotting disorder
   c) canine distemper
   d) infectious canine hepatitis.

126) Sylvatic rabies is the spread of rabies into
   a) domestic dogs and cats
   b) man
   c) non-carnivorous species (e.g. cows)
   d) wildlife.

127) The drug group of choice in the treatment of feline pneumonitis and feline infectious anaemia is
   a) the cephalosporins
   b) the penicillins
   c) the tetracyclines
   d) tylosin.

128) The incubation period for canine distemper is
   a) 1–3 days
   b) 5–7 days
   c) 7–21 days
   d) 21–28 days.

129) There are several clinical signs that are common to both feline rhinotracheitis and feline calicivirus. Which ONE of the following symptoms is MORE common in cases of feline calicivirus infection?
   a) Conjunctivitis
   b) Depression
   c) Sneezing
   d) Tongue ulcers.

130) Which ONE of the following cat diseases is caused by a lentivirus?
  a) FeLV
  b) FIE *(Panleucopenia)*
  c) FIV
  d) FURD.

131) Which ONE of the following dogs is likely to be infected with canine distemper?
  a) The dog has a cough and greenish purulent oculo-nasal discharge
  b) The dog has a cough, but no temperature
  c) The dog has a temperature of 103 deg F (39.4 deg C) and has vomited a number of times
  d) All of the above.

132) Which ONE of the following ectoparasites commonly acts as a vector for a viral disease?
  a) *Cheyletiella*
  b) *Demodex canis*
  c) *Sarcoptes scabiei*
  d) *Spilopsyllus cuniculi.*

133) Which ONE of the following is an example of an adjuvant?
  a) Aluminium hydroxide
  b) Ferrous sulphate
  c) Sodium chloride
  d) Sterile water.

134) Which ONE of the following statements about canine distemper is the MOST accurate?
  a) At least 50% of recovered cases of distemper develop nervous signs later in life
  b) Distemper never occurs as a sub-clinical or mild disease
  c) Dogs that contract distemper usually either die in the early stages , or recover within two or three weeks
  d) Nervous signs due to CDV are mainly seen in dogs which have contracted distemper in old age.

27

135) Which ONE of the following statements concerning FIV infection is NOT true?
   a) The disease is three times more common in females than in males
   b) The disease is rarely seen in cats under one year old
   c) The virus was discovered as recently as 1986
   d) Unlike FeLV, where the virus may be eliminated after the development of an immune response, FIV persists in the body after infection.

136) Which ONE of the following statements is NOT true?
   a) A toxoid is an inactivated vaccine produced by heat-treating a toxin
   b) An anti-toxin is a vaccine against a disease caused by a toxin-producing bacterium, such as tetanus
   c) An autogenous vaccine is a vaccine made from material collected from an animal for administration to the same animal
   d) Mineral oils may be used as adjuvants in inactivated vaccines.

137) Which ONE of the following statements is NOT true?
   a) Once the rabies virus has entered nervous tissue, even at the periphery of the body, vaccination cannot stop the course of the disease
   b) Rabies can affect all mammals, and also birds, as they are all warm blooded
   c) The incubation period for rabies depends on the site of the bite
   d) Vaccination of man after exposure to rabies can be effective in preventing the disease.

138) Which ONE of the following statements is the MOST accurate?
   a) Vaccination against ICH with killed CAV-1 gives good protection against both ICH and respiratory disease
   b) Vaccination against ICH with live, attenuated CAV-1 gives no protection against respiratory disease
   c) Vaccination against ICH with live, attenuated CAV-1 has been superseded by CAV-2 to avoid the risk of *Blue-eye* (corneal oedema)
   d) Vaccination against ICH with live, attenuated CAV-2 has been.

Warning: illegal if copied

139) Which ONE of the following diseases in cats is caused by a herpes virus?

    a) Feline enteritis
    b) Feline leukaemia
    c) Feline rhino-tracheitis
    d) FIV.

140) Which ONE of the following statements is NOT true?

    a) Adenoviruses are quite resistant to drying, and may survive in the environment for up to ten days
    b) Corneal oedema or *Blue Eye* only occurs after vaccination against ICH, never in disease cases
    c) Dogs that have recovered from adenovirus infection may excrete virus for as long as six months
    d) Most cases of *Blue Eye* resolve within a few weeks, but in some cases there is permanent damage to the eye.

141) Which ONE of the following statements is NOT true?

    a) Dogs infected by leptospira may shed organisms for several weeks after recovery
    b) *L. icterohaemorrhagiae* primarily invades the kidney, where it causes tubule cell death
    c) *Leptospira* organisms are readily destroyed by U-V light
    d) *Leptospira* organisms may enter the body through intact mucous membranes.

Other Medical Conditions

142) A *vascular ring defect* occurs where

    a) during embryological development the right aortic arch persists instead of the left, so that after birth the ligamentum arteriosum (the remains of the ductus arteriosus) lies across the oesophagus and interferes with the passage of solids down the oesophagus
    b) the ductus arteriosus persists and remains patent after birth
    c) the foramen ovale — the hole between the two atria — persists after birth
    d) both the foramen ovale and the ductus arteriosus persist after birth.

143) A bitch with diabetes mellitus requires daily insulin (100 iu/ml). She is stable on 20 units per day. What volume would you administer?

 a) 0.025 ml
 b) 0.2 ml
 c) 0.25 ml
 d) 2 ml.

144) A decrease in the number of lymphocytes in the circulation is known as

 a) leukaemia
 b) lymphocytosis
 c) lymphoma
 d) lymphopaenia.

145) A dog exhibiting melaena is most likely to be suffering from

 a) an obstruction at the pylorus
 b) colitis
 c) diarrhoea originating in the large intestine
 d) diarrhoea originating in the small intestine.

146) A three year old, 35 kg German Shepherd dog is admitted because of prolonged seizure activity, and is continuing to fit. Which ONE of the following is the most common consequence of prolonged seizure activity?

 a) Hyperthermia
 b) Liver failure
 c) Permanent blindness
 d) Pneumonia.

147) Addison's disease is also known as

 a) hyperadrenocorticalism
 b) hyperkalaemia
 c) hypoadrenocorticalism
 d) pituitary adenocarcinoma.

148) Atopic dermatitis is
  a) a contact dermatitis caused by allergy to a synthetic substance such as nylon carpets or plastic food bowls
  b) a contact dermatitis caused by an irritant chemical used as a household cleanser
  c) a food hypersensitivity
  d) caused by a wide variety of inhaled environmental allergens, such as house dust mite and pollen.

149) Azotaemia is defined as
  a) an inability to concentrate urine
  b) an increase in the waste nitrogen level in the circulation
  c) high plasma protein levels
  d) hypoproteinaemia.

150) Bedlington terriers can suffer from a defect in hepatic metabolism of which of the following elements?
  a) Calcium
  b) Copper
  c) Manganese
  d) Zinc.

151) Biotin deficiency may be seen in animals
  a) fed a vegetarian diet
  b) fed an entirely muscle-meat diet
  c) fed entirely on liver
  d) fed large numbers of eggs.

152) Cushing's disease is caused by the overproduction of
  a) glucocorticoids
  b) mineralocorticoids
  c) sex steroids
  d) thyroid hormones.

153) Diabetes insipidus is caused by
  a) a failure in the production of aldosterone
  b) a failure in the production of vasopressin
  c) excessive production of aldosterone
  d) excessive production of vasopressin.

154) Endocardiosis is a condition that affects the
   a) body of the stomach
   b) lining of the uterus
   c) valves of the heart
   d) ventricles of the brain.

155) Hypervitaminosis A is *commonly* seen in
   a) cats fed a diet rich in liver
   b) cats fed exclusively on fish
   c) terrapins fed exclusively on muscle meat
   d) terrapins fed on a dry, pelleted diet.

156) In which ONE of the following breeds is exocrine pancreatic insufficiency inheritable?
   a) Bedlington Terriers
   b) Dachshunds
   c) German Shepherd dogs
   d) West Highland White Terriers.

157) In which ONE of the following conditions does glycosuria NOT occur?
   a) Diabetes mellitus
   b) Malabsorption syndrome
   c) Stress
   d) Sudden overconsumption of short chain carbohydrates.

158) Jaundice caused by the excessive breakdown of red blood cells is described as
   a) hepatic jaundice
   b) posthepatic jaundice
   c) prehepatic jaundice
   d) any of the above.

159) Ketoacidosis occurs in diabetes mellitus as a result of
   a) high plasma glucose
   b) low plasma glucose
   c) overdose with insulin
   d) the use of fat as an energy source.

160) Melaena is
    a) blood in the faeces
    b) blood in the urine
    c) blood in the vomit
    d) difficulty passing faeces.

161) Secondary renal hyperparathyroidism is caused by over-activity of the parathyroid gland, which in turn is caused by
    a) a failure of the diseases kidneys to activate vitamin D, which in turn affects calcium metabolism
    b) excessive loss of calcium, producing a change in the Ca:P ratio
    c) retention of phosphorus, which adversely affects the Ca:P ratio
    d) all of the above.

162) Stridor is defined as
    a) muscle atrophy leading to reduction in stride length
    b) increased inspiratory noise, often associated with airway obstruction
    c) increased lung sounds associated with pulmonary oedema
    d) unilateral nasal discharge.

163) The healing of damaged liver tissue by the formation of fibrous tissue is called
    a) ascites
    b) cirrhosis
    c) hepatitis
    d) icterus.

164) The symptoms of acute renal failure may include
    a) oliguria, vomiting, oral ulceration
    b) polyuria, polydipsia, low plasma calcium
    c) polyuria, proteinuria, anaemia
    d) proteinuria, ascites, subcutaneous oedema.

165) The symptoms of nephrotic syndrome include
    a) oliguria, vomiting, oral ulceration
    b) polyuria, polydipsia, low plasma calcium
    c) polyuria, proteinuria, anaemia
    d) proteinuria, ascites, subcutaneous oedema.

166) When a dog is treated for congestive heart failure, potassium supplements may be among the drugs prescribed. This is because
   a) increased plasma potassium decreases the plasma sodium level, thus decreasing blood pressure
   b) increased plasma potassium increases the contractility of heart muscle
   c) potassium potentiates the effect of cardiac glycosides
   d) when diuretics are given, increased amounts of potassium are likely to be lost in the urine.

167) Endocardiosis is
   a) a progressive nodular thickening of the heart valves
   b) inflammation of the heart muscle
   c) inflammation of the lining of the heart
   d) the thinning of the heart muscle of the ventricles seen in dilated cardiomyopathy.

168) Which ONE of the following conditions is NOT likely to give rise to bilateral flank alopecia?
   a) Hyperadrenocorticalism
   b) Hypoadrenocorticalism
   c) Hypothyroidism
   d) Sertoli cell tumour.

169) Which ONE of the following dietary regimes is suitable for a patient with chronic renal failure?
   a) Low protein, high carbohydrate
   b) Low protein, low carbohydrate
   c) High protein, high carbohydrate
   d) High protein, low carbohydrate.

170) Which ONE of the following is NOT likely to be used in the control of feline urolithiasis syndrome?
   a) A low magnesium diet
   b) A low protein diet
   c) Antibiotics
   d) Urinary acidifiers.

171)   Which ONE of the following signs is NOT usually seen in right-sided congestive heart failure?
   a) Ascites
   b) Jugular pulse
   c) Pulmonary oedema
   d) Splenomegaly.

172)   Which ONE of the following statements concerning chronic pulmonary osteoarthropathy (otherwise known as hypertrophic osteopathy) is NOT true?
   a) It is also known as Marie's disease
   b) It is characterised by periosteal bone formation in the distal limbs
   c) It is characterised by severe pulmonary oedema
   d) It is often associated with a space-occupying lesion in the thorax.

173)   Which ONE of the following types of crystals tends to form in alkaline urine?
   a) Ammonium urate
   b) Cystine
   c) Oxalate
   d) Struvite.

174)   Which of the following biochemical estimations is MOST likely to be requested when acute liver damage is suspected?
   a) ALT(SGPT)
   b) Bilirubin
   c) Creatinine
   d) Lipase.

175)   Which of the following biochemical estimations is MOST likely to be requested in a suspected case of acute pancreatitis?
   a) ALT(SGPT)
   b) Bilirubin
   c) Creatinine
   d) Lipase.

176) Which of the following diagnostic tests is NOT likely to be performed in the investigation of a case of Cushing's disease?
  a) ACTH test
  b) Dexamethasone suppression test
  c) Plasma cortisol level
  d) Water deprivation test.

177) Which of the following diseases may be characterised by bi-lateral flank alopecia?
  a) Feline endocrine alopecia
  b) Hypothyroidism
  c) Sertoli cell tumour
  d) All of the above.

178) Which type of cystic calculi are common in Dalmatians?
  a) Ammonium urate
  b) Calcium oxalate
  c) Cystine
  d) Struvite.

Poisons

179) A client phones to say that his young cat was playing with a frog in the garden, and is now pawing at its mouth and salivating profusely. What is your response?
  a) It is most likely that the cat has been stung by an insect
  b) It is most likely that the *frog* was in fact a toad, and the cat has received a dose of toad venom, which is secreted from glands in the skin. This is irritant, but not usually dangerous
  c) It is unlikely that the frog has caused the problem — perhaps the cat has got a foreign body stuck at the back of its mouth
  d) Perhaps the cat has eaten the frog and got a bone wedged across the roof of the mouth.

Warning: illegal if copied

180) What drug is used as an antidote in cases of organophosphorus poisoning?

a) Atropine sulphate
b) Calcium edetate (CaEDTA)
c) Ethanol
d) Vitamin K.

181) What is the common active ingredient in slug pellets?

a) Dicoumarin
b) Ethylene glycol
c) Ethylene oxide
d) Metaldehyde.

182) What is the specific antidote to Warfarin poisoning?

a) Atropine sulphate
b) Cytotoxic drug therapy
c) Fluid therapy
d) Vitamin K.

183) Which ONE of the following drugs is NOT an organophosphorus compound?

a) Dichlorvos
b) Lindane (gamma BHC)
c) Fenthion
d) Malathion.

184) Which ONE of the following drugs is the specific antidote in cases of ethylene glycol poisoning?

a) Atropine sulphate
b) Calcium edetate (CaEDTA)
c) Ethanol
d) Vitamin K.

185) Which ONE of the following drugs is the specific antidote in cases of lead poisoning?

a) Atropine sulphate
b) Calcium edetate (CaEDTA)
c) Ethanol
d) Vitamin K.

186) Which ONE of the following is NOT a COMMON sign of ethylene glycol poisoning in the dog?
   a) Dehydration
   b) Diarrhoea
   c) Dyspnoea
   d) Inco-ordination.

187) Which ONE of the following is the LEAST likely to cause lead poisoning if eaten?
   a) Engine coolant
   b) Fishing weights
   c) Linoleum
   d) Old, flaking paint.

188) Which ONE of the following is the specific antidote to metaldehyde poisoning?
   a) Barbiturates
   b) Diazepam
   c) Ethanol
   d) There is no specific antidote to metaldehyde poisoning.

189) Which ONE of the following rodenticides acts by producing hypothermia?
   a) Alphachloralose
   b) Brodifacoum
   c) Cholecalciferol
   d) Difenacoum.

190) Which ONE of the following statements about anticoagulant rodenticides is the MOST accurate?
   a) Because the *second generation* anticoagulant rodenticides have a longer half life, treatment for poisoning must be continued for longer than if a *first generation* anticoagulant had been used
   b) It is not possible for dogs and cats to suffer warfarin poisoning by eating poisoned rodents
   c) *Second generation* anticoagulant rodenticides were developed with decreased toxicity for non-target species
   d) The *first generation* anticoagulant rodenticides usually only require one feed or intake to produce significant toxicity.

191) Which ONE of the following statements about cholecalciferol as a rodenticide is NOT true?

   a) After gastric evacuation, treatment for cholecalciferol poisoning includes vigorous fluid therapy and administration of frusemide to produce a diuresis
   b) Cholecalciferol is also known as vitamin D
   c) Cholecalciferol rarely causes toxicity in dogs or cats
   d) In some cases, cholecalciferol is included in coumarin rodenticides.

192) Which ONE of the following statements about paraquat poisoning is the LEAST accurate?

   a) Although it is an irritant poison, the induction of vomiting is justified in cases of paraquat ingestion
   b) Early signs of paraquat poisoning may include diarrhoea, but renal failure and pulmonary oedema develop in the later stages
   c) Paraquat poisoning is usually fatal, even if very small quantities have been ingested
   d) Prompt gastric lavage and the administration of Fuller's earth will be successful in saving most cases of paraquat poisoning.

193) Which ONE of the following statements concerning theobromine poisoning is NOT true?

   a) Cooking (baker's) chocolate is more toxic than milk chocolate
   b) Fatalities are rare in dogs following theobromine poisoning — most animals make an uneventful recovery
   c) Signs of poisoning may not develop for more than eight hours after ingestion
   d) Signs of theobromine poisoning vary, but may include vomiting and diarrhoea, seizures, or sudden death from heart failure.

Radiography

194) A focused grid has
   a) both parallel and angled lead slats
   b) lead slats parallel to each other
   c) lead slats parallel to each other but getting smaller in size towards the edge of the grid
   d) lead slats that are at right angles to each other.

195) A radiograph requires an exposure of 20 mAs when taken at a film/focal distance of 90 cm without a grid. What exposure will be required if a grid with a grid factor of 4 is used?
   a) 5 mAs
   b) 20 mAs
   c) 40 mAs
   d) 80 mAs.

196) In which ONE of the following positions should a dog be placed following a myelogram?
   a) Head elevated approximately 30 degrees
   b) Normal recovery position
   c) Sternal recumbency
   d) The head lowered below the rest of the body.

197) Rare earth screens should be used with
   a) fast film
   b) slow film
   c) either fast or slow film
   d) neither.

198) The Radiation Protection Supervisor is usually
   a) a member of the practice, who is responsible for radiation safety but need not be present every time the X-ray machine is used
   b) a member of the practice, who is nominally in charge of radiation safety, and must therefore be present at every radiographic examination
   c) a veterinary surgeon who holds a Diploma in Veterinary radiography, and acts as an advisor in matters of radiation safety
   d) an external advisor, who can advise on radiation protection.

199) The filament of an X-ray tube is normally made of
   a) copper
   b) lead
   c) silver
   d) tungsten.

200) The stem of a stationary anode in an X-ray tube is usually made of
   a) copper
   b) lead
   c) silver
   d) tungsten.

201) The target of an X-ray tube is usually made of
   a) copper
   b) lead
   c) silver
   d) tungsten.

202) What may cause a film to be too pale?
   a) Exhausted developer
   b) Over exposure
   c) Scattered radiation
   d) Static electricity.

203) When positioning a dog for a BVA/KC hip radiograph, the beam should be centred on
   a) the acetabula
   b) the pubic symphysis
   c) the sacrum
   d) the wings of the ilium.

204) When taking a radiograph for the BVA/KC hip displasia scoring scheme, what information must be included on the radiograph?
   a) Dog's name, KC number, L/R marker
   b) KC number, date, L/R marker
   c) KC number, L/R marker
   d) Practice name and address, dog's name, L/R marker.

205) When taking a ventro-dorsal radiograph of the cervical spine, the disc spaces will be viewed most accurately if
   a) the forelimbs are pulled forwards, towards the animal's head
   b) the neck is supported with sandbags
   c) the tube head is inclined 15–20 degrees towards the head
   d) the tube head is inclined 15–20 degrees towards the thorax.

206) Which ONE of the following chemicals is NOT a constituent of the fixer?
   a) Ammonium thiosulphate
   b) Boric acid
   c) Potassium bromide
   d) Sodium acetate.

207) Which ONE of the following controls the quality or penetrating power of the X-ray beam?
   a) KV
   b) mA
   c) Time of exposure
   d) All of the above.

208) Which ONE of the following will NOT reduce the amount of scattered radiation reaching the film when taking a radiograph of the abdomen of a large dog?
   a) Collimation of the primary beam
   b) Increasing the KV
   c) Use of a grid
   d) Use of a compression band.

209) Which ONE of the following is removed from the film during fixing?
   a) Ammonium thiosulphate
   b) Silver halide
   c) Silver nitrate
   d) Sodium chloride.

210) Which ONE of the following items of equipment will reduce the risk of exposure to the primary beam?
   a) Aluminium filter over the tube window
   b) Light beam diaphragm
   c) Protective clothing
   d) Rare earth screens.

211) Which ONE of the following may cause blurring of the film?
   a) Dirty screens
   b) Insufficient washing
   c) Patient movement
   d) Under development.

212) Which ONE of the following statements concerning positioning for radiography is NOT true?
   a) Exposures of the abdomen should always be taken on inspiration
   b) Exposures of the chest should always be taken on inspiration
   c) The nasal chambers are best viewed using an intra-oral non-screen film pushed as far into the mouth over the tongue as possible
   d) To examine the heart, a dorso-ventral view is more useful than a ventro-dorsal view, as in the latter the heart may tip to one side.

213) Which ONE of the following statements concerning safety during radiography is the LEAST accurate?
   a) A lead-lined apron of standard thickness will protect against scattered radiation, and also against the primary beam, should it be required to do so
   b) Lead lined gloves and shields should never be used in the primary beam, as they do not provide sufficient protection
   c) Manual restraint of an animal should never be undertaken unless the machine is fitted with a light beam diaphragm
   d) To minimise exposure, grids should not be used unless the part being X-rayed is at least 10 cm thick.

214) Which ONE of the following will reduce the amount of scattered radiation reaching the film?
   a) Increasing the film/focal distance
   b) Increasing the KV and decreasing the mA
   c) Reducing the exposure time and increasing the mA
   d) Reducing the size of the primary beam.

215) Which film fault is responsible for white spots on the radiograph?
   a) Dirt on the intensifying screens
   b) Film not agitated sufficiently
   c) Film underdeveloped
   d) Fixer splashed onto the film before processing.

216) Which is the *fixing agent* used in a fixer?
   a) Ammonium chloride
   b) Ammonium thiosulphate
   c) Potassium hydroxide
   d) Sodium acetate.

217) You have developed a radiograph using the wet tank method, and the film has turned out yellow. What is this due to?
   a) Contamination of the developer
   b) Exhausted developer
   c) Fixer being spilt on the film before processing
   d) Fixing time too short.

Surgical Nursing

General Surgical Nursing

218) A cold abscess is
   a) an abscess that drains to an epithelial surface via a sinus tract
   b) an abscess that has not yet come to a head
   c) an abscess that forms without causing noticeable inflammation of the surrounding tissue
   d) where the abscess cavity is lined with a thick, fibrous wall, enclosing a cavity full of necrotic debris, but no live bacteria.

Warning: illegal if copied

44

219) A comminuted fracture is one where
   a) the joint is involved in the fracture
   b) the skin overlying the fracture is broken and bone ends protrude
   c) the two fractured ends of bone have moved past each other
   d) there are more than two fracture fragments.

220) A localised accumulation of dead and viable neutrophils in a cavity lined with fibrous tissue is called
   a) an abscess
   b) cellulitis
   c) a cyst
   d) an ulcer.

221) A papilloma is a
   a) benign tumour of adipose tissue, common in the subcutis of older dogs
   b) benign tumour of fibrous tissue
   c) benign tumour of the epithelial melanocytes
   d) benign, wart-like tumour of epithelial cells.

222) A plaster cast applied in order to immobilise a mid-shaft fracture of the radius should extend from
   a) above the elbow, and include the whole foot
   b) above the elbow to below the carpus
   c) just below the elbow to just above the carpus
   d) the shoulder to the metacarpus.

223) A sutured operative wound in the oral mucosa is defined as
   a) a clean-contaminated wound
   b) a clean wound
   c) a contaminated wound
   d) an infected wound.

224) A temporary tracheotomy tube should be cleaned to remove accumulated mucus
   a) daily
   b) two or three times daily
   c) every two to three hours
   d) every hour.

225) Although to a large extent superseded by internal fixation techniques, Schroeder-Thomas extension splints are still used from time to time. In which ONE of the following circumstances might such a splint be used?
   a) A fracture of the calcaneus
   b) A fracture of the radius and ulna
   c) A fracture of three metatarsal bones
   d) A transverse fracture of the distal third of the femur.

226) An allograft is a skin graft that
   a) has come from a different animal of the same species
   b) has come from an animal of a different species
   c) has come from elsewhere on the same animal
   d) includes only the epidermis and a small sliver of dermis.

227) An inflammatory reaction where pus is distributed through cleavage planes and tissue spaces is called
   a) a cold abscess
   b) an abscess
   c) cellulitis
   d) ulceration.

228) Anal furunculosis is MOST commonly seen in
   a) Cavalier King Charles spaniels
   b) German shepherd dogs
   c) Labrador retrievers
   d) Pekingese.

229) Dehiscence is defined as
   a) poor blood supply to a wound caused by bruising of the surrounding tissues
   b) skin necrosis caused by excessively tight sutures
   c) the formation of a seroma on the site of a surgical wound
   d) wound breakdown.

230) During fracture fixation, a previously tapped hole is used with a

 a) compression plate and screws
 b) Venables plate and screws
 c) Rush plate and screws
 d) Sherman plate and screws.

231) For which ONE of the following reasons may a veterinary surgeon perform a cystotomy?

 a) To dissect out a portion of the bladder wall due to a tumour
 b) To remove bladder stones
 c) To unblock the urethra if urinary calculi are causing a blockage
 d) None of the above.

232) Fracture disease is

 a) another term for mal-union of a fracture
 b) osteomyelitis following an open fracture
 c) rigidity of one or more joints in a limb following fracture repair
 d) the shortening of a limb following the repair of a fracture.

233) How is the stifle joint MOST commonly supported post-operatively?

 a) A plaster backslab
 b) A plaster cylinder
 c) A Robert Jones bandage
 d) A Thomas splint.

234) In an emergency tracheotomy, performed because of acute and near-complete upper airway obstruction, and without a veterinary surgeon being on the premises, the nurse should
   a) clip and prepare the skin before incising carefully just behind the larynx
   b) having incised the skin and separated the muscles in the ventral midline make a vertical incision through two or three tracheal rings
   c) wait until he/she can contact a veterinary surgeon before performing the surgical procedure
   d) without wasting time on skin preparation, and having incised the skin and separated the muscles in the ventral midline, make an incision between the second and third tracheal cartilages.

235) In the management of large wounds carrying a significant amount of black necrotic tissue, the aim must be to encourage this necrotic tissue to slough. Which ONE of the following dressings is NOT appropriate for this task?
   a) A dry non-adherent dressing
   b) An alginate dressing
   c) An occlusive hydrocolloid dressing
   d) Successive wet packs made up with sterile saline.

236) In the process of wound healing, organisation is defined as
   a) the process by which inflammatory tissue is removed once an abscess is drained
   b) the replacement of damaged tissue by scar tissue
   c) the replacement of destroyed tissue by similar functional tissue
   d) the return of the tissue to the state it was in before the start of the inflammatory process.

237) Kirschner wires differ from Steinman pins in that
   a) the Kirschner wire is a thin version of the Steinman pin
   b) there is no difference between them
   c) they are curved pins, rather than straight
   d) they have a flattened instead of a trocar point.

238) Rongeurs are
   a) a self-retaining retractor
   b) a type of dental elevator
   c) haemostats
   d) designed for nibbling away small pieces of bone.

239) The accumulation of debris as a film covering the teeth, made up of bacteria, food particles and saliva is known as
   a) dental calculus
   b) gingivitis
   c) plaque
   d) tartar.

240) The callus that forms at the site of a fracture is made up of
   a) cartilage
   b) fibrous tissue, cartilage and immature bone
   c) remains of a blood clot, plus fibrous tissue
   d) remodelled new bone which completes the fracture repair.

241) The correct suffix for a term describing the surgical removal of all or part of a structure is
   a) -ectomy
   b) -itis
   c) -ostomy
   d) -otomy.

242) The scaling of teeth should not be performed at the same time as other major surgery because
   a) different antibiotics may be required for the two different procedures
   b) it increases the time the animal is under general anaesthetic, and therefore increases the anaesthetic risk
   c) scaling can produce oral discomfort for some days afterwards, so the patient is less willing to eat, and takes longer to recover from surgery
   d) scaling releases bacteria from the mouth into the bloodstream, leading to a increased risk of wound infection.

49

243) The term *transplantation* describes tumour spread
  a) by direct invasion of neighbouring tissue
  b) by the shedding of tumour cells into a body cavity
  c) via the bloodstream
  d) via the lymphatic system.

244) What is the name of the technique whereby a needle is put through the abdominal wall in order to drain urine from the bladder?
  a) Abdominocentesis
  b) Cystocentesis
  c) Percutaneous compression
  d) Thoracocentesis.

245) What type of skin graft is made up of small plugs of dermis which are implanted in matching holes cut in the bed of granulation tissue?
  a) Mesh graft
  b) Pinch graft
  c) Stamp graft
  d) Strip graft.

246) Which ONE of the following is NOT a disadvantage in the use of drains in surgical wounds?
  a) Drains may allow infection to gain access to the body
  b) The animal must be prevented from trying to remove the drain — often by wearing an Elizabethan collar
  c) The presence of a drain will usually increase the time taken for the original surgical wound to heal
  d) They act as foreign bodies within the tissues.

247) Which ONE of the following is NOT a property of the synthetic casting materials, eg. Vetcast, in comparison to Plaster of Paris?
  a) Cheaper
  b) Radiolucent
  c) Stronger
  d) Water resistant.

248) Which ONE of the following is NOT often a feature of malignant tumours?

 a) Encapsulation
 b) Haemorrhage
 c) Irregular shape
 d) Ulceration.

249) Which ONE of the following precautions is the LEAST use in the prevention of hypothermia in small mammals during surgery?

 a) During skin preparation, wet the skin of the animal as little as possible, using surgical spirit only if absolutely necessary
 b) Give warmed fluids subcutaneously post-operatively
 c) Make sure the ambient temperature in the operating theatre is kept quite high
 d) Use a heat pad under the animal throughout the surgical procedure.

250) Which ONE of the following signs is NOT usually indicative of hypothermia?

 a) Cold extremities
 b) Increased heart rate
 c) Pale mucous membranes
 d) Relative inactivity.

251) Which ONE of the following types of retractor are self-retaining?

 a) Gelpi
 b) Hohman
 c) Langenbeck
 d) All of the above.

Anaesthesia

252) 90% of the soda lime used in a Water's canister is made up of
 a) calcium carbonate
 b) calcium hydroxide
 c) calcium oxalate
 d) calcium sulphate.

51

253) A 30 kg dog is anaesthetised, and maintained on a Magill circuit. What flow rate will be required if the dog is breathing about 20 times a minute?
   a) 3–5 litres/minute
   b) 6–8 litres/minute
   c) 9–11 litres/minute
   d) 12–14 litres/minute.

254) A Magill circuit can be classified as which type of anaesthetic circuit?
   a) Open
   b) Closed
   c) Semi-open
   d) Semi-closed.

255) A Circle circuit can be classified as which type of anaesthetic circuit?
   a) Open
   b) Closed
   c) Semi-open
   d) Semi-closed.

256) A standard Bain circuit may be altered to form a modified Bain circuit by
   a) having a valve on the expiratory limb, and a closed reservoir bag
   b) having an open-ended bag on the expiratory limb
   c) moving the reservoir bag to the inspiratory limb
   d) using parallel rather than co-axial tubing.

257) Adrenaline is included in bottles of local anaesthetic for use by local infiltration for the following reason.
   a) It aids the absorption of the lignocaine into the CNS
   b) It aids the rapid dispersal of the drug throughout the body
   c) It causes local vasoconstriction, keeping the drug where it is placed for a longer period of time
   d) It reduces the likelihood of a decrease in heart rate due to the effect of the lignocaine.

258) An ataractic drug produces
   a) a calming and sedative effect
   b) a decrease in saliva production
   c) an increase in excitability
   d) an increase in heart rate.

259) Calculate the flow rates required of oxygen and nitrous oxide for a 15 kg dog to be maintained on a Lack circuit (assuming a minute volume of 200 ml/kg).
   a) 1 litre oxygen, 2 litres nitrous oxide
   b) 1.5 litres oxygen, 2.5 litres nitrous oxide
   c) 2.5 litres oxygen, 5 litres nitrous oxide
   d) 3.5 litres oxygen, 6.5 litres nitrous oxide.

260) Calculate the flow rates required of oxygen and nitrous oxide for a 25 kg dog to be maintained on a Magill circuit (assuming a minute volume of 200 ml/kg)
   a) 1.25 litres oxygen, 2.5 litres nitrous oxide
   b) 1.75 litres oxygen, 3.25 litres nitrous oxide
   c) 2.25 litres oxygen, 4.5 litres nitrous oxide
   d) 2.75 litres oxygen, 5.5 litres nitrous oxide.

261) Calculate the flow rates required of oxygen and nitrous oxide for a 8 kg dog to be maintained on a Ayres T-piece circuit (assuming a minute volume of 200 ml/kg).
   a) 1 litre oxygen, 2 litres nitrous oxide
   b) 1.5 litres oxygen, 2.5 litres nitrous oxide
   c) 2.5 litres oxygen, 5 litres nitrous oxide
   d) 3.5 litres oxygen, 6.5 litres nitrous oxide.

262) Calculate the volume of *Saffan* (12 mg/ml) required to anaesthetise a cat weighing 6 kg, assuming a dose rate of 3 mg/kg
   a) 1 ml
   b) 1.5 ml
   c) 2 ml
   d) 2.5 ml.

263) Calculate the volume of 1.25% thiopentone required to anaesthetise a 3.75 kg cat, assuming a dose rate of 10 mg/kg
   a) 2 ml
   b) 3 ml
   c) 4 ml
   d) 5 ml.

264) Calculate the volume of 2.5% thiopentone required to anaesthetise a 25 kg labrador, assuming a dose rate of 10 mg/kg.
   a) 10 ml
   b) 15 ml
   c) 20 ml
   d) 30 ml.

265) Central venous pressure is measured in the
   a) left atrium
   b) left ventricle
   c) right atrium
   d) right ventricle.

266) External cardio-pulmonary resuscitation carried out by ONE
person should be as follows:
   a) 1 cardiac compression, 5 breaths
   b) 5 cardiac compressions, 1 breath
   c) 2 cardiac compressions, 15 breaths
   d) 15 cardiac compressions, 2 breaths.

267) Glycopyrrolate is
   a) a non-steroidal anti-inflammatory
   b) a tranquilliser
   c) an antipyretic
   d) an antisialogogue.

268) How much anaesthetic agent is there in 100 ml of a 5%
solution?
   a) 5 mg
   b) 50 mg
   c) 500 mg
   d) 5000 mg.

269) Identify the following anaesthetic circuit.

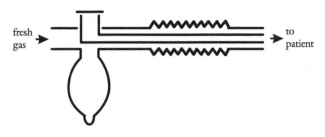

fresh gas → to patient

a) Ayres T-piece (Jackson-Rees modification)
b) Bain
c) Lack
d) Magill.

270) Identify the following anaesthetic circuit.

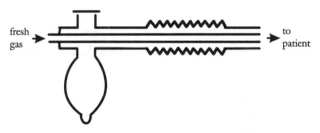

fresh gas → to patient

a) Ayres T-piece (Jackson-Rees modification)
b) Bain
c) Lack
d) Magill.

271) Identify the following anaesthetic circuit.

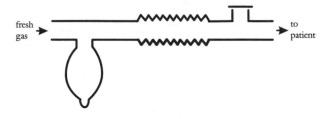

a) Ayres T-piece (Jackson-Rees modification.)
b) Bain
c) Lack
d) Magill.

272) Identify the following anaesthetic circuit.

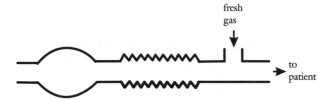

a) Ayres T-piece (Jackson-Rees modification)
b) Bain
c) Lack
d) Magill.

273) In exhausted soda lime, all the active salt has been converted to
a) calcium carbonate
b) calcium hydroxide
c) calcium oxalate
d) calcium sulphate.

274) Nitrous oxide is contained in cylinders that are
   a) black with a white neck
   b) blue
   c) grey
   d) orange.

275) Open, part-used vials of *Saffan* should NOT be stored in the refrigerator because
   a) intravenous injection of cold fluids may harm the patient
   b) the various constituent drugs precipitate out at low temperatures
   c) they contain a preservative, so will not deteriorate at room temperature
   d) they contain a bacteriostat, so can be stored at room temperature.

276) Open, part-used vials of *Propofol* should be stored
   a) at room temperature for up to 48 hours
   b) in the refrigerator for up to 24 hours
   c) in the refrigerator for up to 7 days
   d) part used vials of propofol should be discarded at the end of the day.

277) Oxygen is supplied in cylinders that are
   a) black with a white neck
   b) blue
   c) grey
   d) orange.

278) Part-used containers of soda lime should be kept tightly sealed
   a) because soda lime is highly inflammable
   b) to prevent the atmospheric carbon dioxide exhausting the soda lime
   c) to prevent water absorption by the granules
   d) to stop accidental inhalation of the fine dust.

279) The first step in cardio-pulmonary resuscitation is to
   a) begin external chest compressions
   b) establish an airway
   c) give adrenaline
   d) ventilate with 100% oxygen.

280) The minute volume for all mammals may be considered to be approximately
   a) 20 ml/kg/minute
   b) 50 ml/kg/minute
   c) 100 ml/kg/minute
   d) 200 ml/kg/minute.

281) The occasional anaphylactoid reactions seen in cats following injection of *Saffan* are due to
   a) anaesthetic overdose
   b) perivascular injection of the anaesthetic
   c) reaction to alphaxolone
   d) reaction to Cremophor EL.

282) The statement *this drug has a very high therapeutic index* means that
   a) it is very easy to overdose using this drug
   b) this drug can be given at several times its recommended dose rate with relative safety
   c) this drug is very effective at its recommended dose rate
   d) this drug may cause excitement on administration.

283) When should the endotracheal tube be removed from a cat, following surgery?
   a) As soon as surgery is finished
   b) It should be left in place as long as possible
   c) Just after the swallowing reflex returns
   d) Just before the swallowing reflex returns.

284) Which ONE of the following anaesthetic circuits should NOT normally be used with nitrous oxide?
 a) Ayres's T-piece
 b) Bain
 c) Closed to-and-fro
 d) Magill.

285) Which ONE of the following drugs is NOT a muscle relaxant?
 a) Edrophonium
 b) Pancuronium
 c) Succinylcholine
 d) Vecuronium.

286) Which ONE of the following drugs is a benzodiazepine?
 a) Acepromazine
 b) Buprenorphine
 c) Diazepam
 d) Ketamine.

287) Which ONE of the following drugs is a dissociative anaesthetic?
 a) Acepromazine
 b) Buprenorphine
 c) Diazepam
 d) Ketamine.

288) Which ONE of the following drugs is a phenothiazine?
 a) Acepromazine
 b) Buprenorphine
 c) Diazepam
 d) Ketamine.

289) Which ONE of the following drugs is an antisialogogue?
 a) Glycopyrrolate
 b) Midezolam
 c) Pentazocine
 d) Suxamethonium.

290) Which ONE of the following drugs is an opioid analgesic?
a) Acepromazine
b) Buprenorphine
c) Diazepam
d) Ketamine.

291) Which ONE of the following is NOT a controlled drug?
a) Buprenorphine
b) Morphine
c) Pentobarbitone
d) Propofol.

292) Which ONE of the following is NOT a potential hazard to personnel who are in the operating theatre when a volatile anaesthetic is in use?
a) Brain tumour
b) Complication of pregnancy
c) Explosion
d) Liver damage.

293) Which ONE of the following is NOT a property of acepromazine?
a) It is antiemetic
b) It is contraindicated in dyspnoeic patients
c) It is contraindicated in epileptic patients
d) It is hypertensive.

294) Which ONE of the following is a property of nitrous oxide?
a) It causes significant respiratory depression
b) It does not require scavenging
c) It is an analgesic
d) It is explosive.

295) Which ONE of the following is a schedule 2 controlled drug?
a) Buprenorphine
b) Morphine
c) Pentobarbitone
d) Phenobarbitone.

296) Which ONE of the following is a schedule 3 controlled drug?
a) Buprenorphine
b) Diazepam
c) Etorphine
d) Pethidine.

297) Which ONE of the following statements about Boyle's bottle and its use is the LEAST accurate?
a) Ambient temperature will affect the concentration of anaesthetic delivered
b) As the liquid anaesthetic vaporises, the remaining liquid cools
c) Boyle's bottle must ONLY be used with oxygen, never with an oxygen/nitrous oxide mixture
d) During the course of an anaesthetic, without adjustment of the plunger, the concentration of delivered anaesthetic will gradually fall.

298) Which ONE of the following statements about ketamine is NOT true?
a) Ketamine produces minimal cardiovascular and respiratory depression
b) Ketamine gives good analgesia
c) Ketamine gives good muscle relaxation
d) Ketamine tends to preserve the cough reflex.

299) Which ONE of the following statements about methohexitone is NOT true?
a) Animals make a much faster recovery from methohexitone than from thiopentone
b) It is much faster acting than thiopentone
c) It is twice as potent as thiopentone
d) Perivascular injection does not cause tissue damage as does thiopentone.

300) Which ONE of the following statements about *Propofol* is
      NOT true?
      a) It causes less respiratory depression than thiopentone
      b) It is non-cumulative when administered by infusion in dogs
      c) It often causes a transient apnoea on induction
      d) It should not be stored once the vial has been opened.

301) Which ONE of the following statements about minute vol-
      ume is the MOST accurate?
      a) Although there is a standard number for the minute volume
           of all animals, generally speaking, the heavier animals have a
           larger minute volume
      b) Although there is a standard number for the minute volume
           of all animals, generally speaking, the smaller animals have a
           larger minute volume
      c) The minute volume varies according to the anaesthetic drugs
           that are being used
      d) The minute volume varies according to the anaesthetic system
           that is being used.

302) Which ONE of the following statements about opioid anal-
      gesics is NOT true?
      a) In pain-free animals, opioids may produce stimulation rather
           than sedation
      b) Morphine often causes vomiting in dogs
      c) Opioid analgesics tend to increase heart rate
      d) Prolonged use of opioid analgesics tends to cause constipation.

303) Which ONE of the following statements is NOT true?
      a) Bradycardia is often seen as a response to pain
      b) Bradycardia, unless it is excessive, increases ventricular filling
           and reduces the work the heart has to do to pump blood
      c) Tachycardia is caused by adrenaline release
      d) Tachycardia is desirable as a physiological response to
           hypotension.

304) Which ONE of the following statements is NOT true?
a) *Hypnorm* is a commercially produced neuroleptanalgesic
b) Neuroleptanalgesia is the combination of a potent tranquilliser and an analgesic
c) Neuroleptanalgesia produces profound anaesthesia by intravenous injection without cardiac or respiratory depression
d) The antidote to etorphine in man is naloxone.

305) Which ONE of the following statements is true?
a) Nitrous oxide is supplied as a compressed gas in blue cylinders
b) Nitrous oxide is supplied as a compressed liquid in grey cylinders
c) Oxygen is supplied as a compressed gas in cylinders that are black with a white top
d) Oxygen is supplied as a compressed gas in cylinders that are white with a black top.

306) Which ONE of the following statements is true?
a) An increase in respiratory rate may be seen in deeply anaesthetised animals
b) Heart rate is a good indicator of anaesthetic depth
c) Most anaesthetic agents tend to increase blood pressure
d) Pulse rate is a good indicator of blood pressure.

307) Which of the following flow rates of oxygen and nitrous oxide would you use for a 20 kg dog to be maintained on a Bain circuit?
a) 1 litre oxygen; 2 litres nitrous oxide
b) 1.5 litres oxygen; 2.5 litres nitrous oxide
c) 2.5 litres oxygen; 5 litres nitrous oxide
d) 3.5 litres oxygen; 6.5 litres nitrous oxide.

308) Which of the following is NOT a DISADVANTAGE of using a Waters canister in a closed, to-and-fro anaesthetic circuit?
  a) Care must be taken to completely fill the canister, or all the carbon dioxide will not be absorbed
  b) Particles of soda lime may be inhaled by the patient
  c) The canister is large and unwieldy, yet needs to be close to the patient to minimise dead space
  d) The cost of replacing the soda lime adds significantly to the cost of the anaesthetic.

309) Which ONE of the following is unlikely to be a cause of cardiac arrest under anaesthesia?
  a) Anaesthetic overdose
  b) Hyperventilation
  c) Hypotension
  d) Toxaemia.

310) You are asked to prepare a syringe containing enough thiopentone to induce anaesthesia in a 35 kg labrador. The dose required is 10 mg/kg. You have a 2.5% solution. What volume would you use?
  a) 1.4 ml
  b) 7 ml
  c) 14 ml
  d) 17 ml.

Theatre Practice

311) *Chromic* catgut has been treated with chromium salts in order to
  a) increase its shelf life
  b) make it less irritant to tissues
  c) make it less likely to break when knots are tied
  d) to slow down the rate of breakdown in the body.

312) A hand scrub using pevidine should be performed for
   a) 1–2 minutes
   b) 3–5 minutes
   c) 5–10 minutes
   d) 15 minutes.

313) A hot air oven sterilises at
   a) 121 deg C
   b) 126 deg C
   c) 135 deg C
   d) over 150 deg C.

314) Ethylene oxide is MOST commonly used to sterilise articles that
   a) are made of PVC (polyvinylchloride)
   b) cannot be dried effectively
   c) need to be sterilised quickly
   d) tend to be damaged by heat.

315) Glove powder is made of
   a) antibiotic powder
   b) maize starch
   c) sodium bicarbonate
   d) talcum powder.

316) In what type of surgical procedure would you be MOST likely to use a periosteal elevator?
   a) Abdominal
   b) Diaphragmatic
   c) Ophthalmic
   d) Orthopaedic.

317) The disadvantage of using spore strips to check for effective sterilisation is that
 a) they only check for spores, not viruses or bacteria
 b) they only indicate the temperature reached, not how long it was maintained
 c) they only work in an autoclave
 d) they require incubation after exposure, so the results aren't known for several days.

318) The surgical gown should be folded before sterilisation so that which part of the gown is uppermost when the pack is opened?
 a) The cuffs of the gown sleeves
 b) The inside of the gown shoulder seams
 c) The inside of the gown waist seam
 d) The outside of the gown waist.

319) What is a Volkmann's spoon?
 a) A curette
 b) A lobe in the cerebellum of the brain
 c) An indentation of the pelvis
 d) An instrument used to dispense powders or granules.

320) What is the function of Spencer Wells forceps?
 a) Haemostasis
 b) Muscle retraction
 c) Needle holders
 d) Tissue forceps.

321) What is the name of the needle holder used in ophthalmic surgical procedures?
 a) Castroviejo's
 b) Debakey's
 c) Kilner's
 d) Mayo Hagar's.

Warning: illegal if copied

322) What type of needle should be used on delicate soft tissue?
a) A curved cutting needle
b) A round bodied needle
c) A straight cutting needle
d) A taper-cut needle.

323) When draping a prepared surgical site (e.g. an abdomen for laparotomy), the first drape to be positioned should be the one
a) between the surgeon and the patient
b) nearest the head of the patient
c) nearest the tail of the patient
d) the furthest from the surgeon.

324) When putting on surgical gloves before major surgery, which ONE of the following methods is recommended?
a) Closed gloving
b) Open gloving
c) Overgloving
d) Plunge gloving.

325) When using a Browne's tube, what colour indicates that the correct temperature has been maintained for the correct time?
a) Blue
b) Brown
c) Green
d) Orange.

326) Where should the earthplate of a diathermy machine be placed when in use?
a) Between the patient and the drapes
b) Between the patient and the rubber table top
c) Between the rubber table top and the table
d) On the floor beneath the table.

327) Which ONE of the following is NOT an essential precaution when using liquid nitrogen as a refrigerant in cryosurgery?
   a) Make sure the stopper is always firmly screwed down on the container when not in use
   b) Take care not to touch metal instruments that have been pre-cooled in contact with liquid nitrogen
   c) Use protective eye goggles
   d) Wear well-insulated gloves to avoid splashing liquid nitrogen on the hands.

328) Which ONE of the following should NOT be included in the daily cleaning routine for an operating theatre?
   a) All cleaning utensils should be used only in the operating theatre, not in other parts of the hospital
   b) At the beginning of the day, wipe over all surfaces with a dry cloth
   c) At the end of the day, any loose hair and debris should be vacuumed up before washing the floor
   d) Between operations, the operating table and any soiled surfaces should be wiped clean.

329) Which ONE of the following skin preparations should be used prior to surgery round the eye or on oral mucosa?
   a) Chlorhexidine
   b) Povidine iodine
   c) Surgical spirit
   d) Either a or b.

330) Which ONE of the following suture materials is NOT absorbable?
   a) Catgut
   b) Polydioxanone
   c) Polyglactin 910
   d) Polypropylene.

Warning: illegal if copied

331) Which ONE of the following types of forceps is a bowel clamp?
  a) Adson's
  b) Cheatle
  c) Doyen
  d) Gillies.

332) Which ONE of the following will NOT reduce the effectiveness of autoclaving as a means of sterilisation of surgical packs?
  a) Dried blood left on instruments
  b) Overloading the autoclave
  c) Stacking packs without space between them
  d) Underfilling the autoclave.

333) Which ONE of the following scalpel blades requires a size 4 scalpel handle?
  a) 10
  b) 11
  c) 15
  d) 20.

334) Why do some surgical instruments have gold coloured handles?
  a) To prevent rusting
  b) To prevent them becoming magnetised
  c) To reduce the build up of static electricity
  d) To show they have tungsten inserts.

335) Why do some swabs have a black line in them?
  a) To indicate their weight and absorbency
  b) To indicate they are not suitable for use in body cavities
  c) To make them easier to see when saturated with blood
  d) To make them visible on X-ray.

Obstetrical and Paediatric Nursing

336) A prospective dam that is nearing delivery should be fed
   a) a fat free diet
   b) a high fibre diet
   c) frequent small meals
   d) b and c.

337) At which stage of parturition is dystocia diagnosed?
   a) First stage
   b) Second stage
   c) Third stage
   d) It may be at any stage.

338) During parturition, which ONE of the fetal membranes must be ruptured before the fetus can move into the birth canal?
   a) Amnion
   b) Allantois
   c) Chorio-allantois
   d) Primitive yolk sac.

339) Pregnant bitches should be wormed during pregnancy
   a) three weeks before parturition
   b) ten days before parturition
   c) a week before parturition
   d) Bitches should not be wormed during pregnancy.

340) The cat is said to be seasonally polyoestrus. This means that
   a) many ova are released during each oestrus cycle
   b) the cat has recurrent oestrus cycles throughout the breeding season
   c) the cat has recurrent oestrus cycles throughout the year
   d) the cat only comes into oestrus during the spring and autumn months.

Warning: illegal if copied

341) The hormone responsible for the maintenance of pregnancy in the bitch is
   a) follicle stimulating hormone
   b) luteinising hormone
   c) oestradiol
   d) progesterone.

342) The normal range of rectal temperature for pups in the first week of life is
   a) 32–34 deg C
   b) 35–37 deg C
   c) 38–40 deg C
   d) 40–42 deg C.

343) The regime for hand-rearing neonatal pups should include feeding
   a) every 1–2 hours for the first five days, reducing to every 4 hours
   b) every 4 hours for the first five days, reducing to every 6 hours
   c) every 2–4 hours for the first five days, reducing to every 4 hours
   d) every 2–4 hours for the first five days, reducing to every 6 hours.

344) The term *primagravida* means
   a) the animal has been mated for the first time
   b) the animal has had its first season
   c) the animal referred to was the first to be born of the litter
   d) the first pregnancy.

345) Ultrasound can be used during pregnancy to
   a) accurately predict the number of puppies in the uterus
   b) determine fetal viability
   c) estimate the stage of fetal development
   d) both b and c.

346) When a pup presents in the birth canal with the rump and tail first and the hindlegs directed towards its head it is termed
   a) a breech presentation
   b) a normal presentation
   c) a posterior presentation
   d) an anterior presentation.

347) Which ONE of the following discharges is normal after kittening?
   a) A dark brown discharge
   b) A heavy green discharge
   c) A white serous discharge
   d) Bloody mucus.

348) Which ONE of the following is NOT a sign of first stage parturition in the bitch?
   a) Hyperthermia
   b) Panting
   c) Presence of milk
   d) Restlessness.

349) Which ONE of the following statements is the MOST accurate?
   a) In a normal bitch, prepartum hyperthermia precedes parturition by 24–36 hours. The temperature may rise by as much as 2 deg C
   b) In a normal bitch, prepartum hypothermia precedes parturition by 24–36 hours. The temperature may drop by as much as 2 deg C
   c) In a normal bitch, prepartum hypothermia precedes parturition by 48–72 hours. The temperature rarely drops more than 1 deg C
   d) Occasionally, prepartum hypothermia precedes parturition by 48–72 hours. The temperature may drop by as much as 2 deg C.

350) Which of the following species is NOT an induced ovulator?
   a) Cat
   b) Ferret
   c) Guinea pig
   d) Rabbit.

Answers

1)	b	27)	c	53)	c	79)	d
2)	b	28)	a	54)	a	80)	b
3)	d	29)	c	55)	b	81)	b
4)	b	30)	a	56)	d	82)	c
5)	b	31)	d	57)	b	83)	b
6)	c	32)	c	58)	b	84)	a
7)	d	33)	a	59)	b	85)	c
8)	b	34)	d	60)	d	86)	d
9)	a	35)	c	61)	d	87)	c
10)	b	36)	a	62)	a	88)	d
11)	c	37)	c	63)	c	89)	d
12)	b	38)	c	64)	c	90)	c
13)	c	39)	d	65)	d	91)	b
14)	d	40)	c	66)	d	92)	c
15)	a	41)	b	67)	c	93)	c
16)	b	42)	b	68)	c	94)	a
17)	c	43)	b	69)	a	95)	b
18)	d	44)	b	70)	b	96)	b
19)	c	45)	a	71)	d	97)	b
20)	b	46)	b	72)	a	98)	a
21)	b	47)	a	73)	b	99)	b
22)	d	48)	a	74)	d	100)	d
23)	c	49)	a	75)	a	101)	c
24)	b	50)	b	76)	a	102)	b
25)	d	51)	a	77)	c	103)	c
26)	b	52)	d	78)	b	104)	a

105)	b	143)	b	181)	d	219)	d
106)	d	144)	d	182)	d	220)	a
107)	b	145)	d	183)	b	221)	d
108)	c	146)	a	184)	c	222)	b
109)	b	147)	c	185)	b	223)	a
110)	c	148)	d	186)	b	224)	c
111)	c	149)	b	187)	a	225)	d
112)	b	150)	b	188)	d	226)	a
113)	b	151)	d	189)	a	227)	c
114)	b	152)	a	190)	a	228)	b
115)	d	153)	b	191)	c	229)	d
116)	b	154)	c	192)	d	230)	a
117)	a	155)	a	193)	b	231)	b
118)	d	156)	c	194)	a	232)	c
119)	a	157)	b	195)	d	233)	c
120)	c	158)	c	196)	a	234)	d
121)	b	159)	d	197)	a	235)	a
122)	c	160)	a	198)	a	236)	b
123)	d	161)	d	199)	d	237)	d
124)	c	162)	b	200)	a	238)	d
125)	d	163)	b	201)	d	239)	c
126)	d	164)	a	202)	a	240)	b
127)	c	165)	d	203)	b	241)	a
128)	c	166)	d	204)	b	242)	d
129)	d	167)	a	205)	c	243)	b
130)	c	168)	b	206)	c	244)	b
131)	a	169)	a	207)	a	245)	b
132)	d	170)	b	208)	b	246)	c
133)	a	171)	c	209)	b	247)	a
134)	a	172)	c	210)	b	248)	a
135)	a	173)	d	211)	c	249)	b
136)	b	174)	a	212)	a	250)	b
137)	b	175)	d	213)	a	251)	a
138)	c	176)	d	214)	d	252)	b
139)	c	177)	d	215)	a	253)	b
140)	b	178)	a	216)	b	254)	d
141)	b	179)	b	217)	d	255)	b
142)	a	180)	a	218)	d	256)	a

257)	c	281)	d	305)	c	329)	b
258)	a	282)	b	306)	a	330)	d
259)	a	283)	d	307)	d	331)	c
260)	b	284)	c	308)	d	332)	d
261)	b	285)	a	309)	b	333)	d
262)	b	286)	c	310)	c	334)	d
263)	b	287)	d	311)	d	335)	d
264)	a	288)	a	312)	c	336)	c
265)	c	289)	a	313)	d	337)	b
266)	d	290)	b	314)	d	338)	c
267)	d	291)	d	315)	b	339)	b
268)	d	292)	a	316)	d	340)	b
269)	c	293)	d	317)	d	341)	d
270)	b	294)	c	318)	b	342)	a
271)	d	295)	b	319)	a	343)	c
272)	a	296)	a	320)	a	344)	d
273)	a	297)	c	321)	a	345)	d
274)	b	298)	c	322)	b	346)	a
275)	b	299)	b	323)	a	347)	a
276)	d	300)	a	324)	a	348)	a
277)	a	301)	b	325)	c	349)	b
278)	b	302)	c	326)	b	350)	c
279)	b	303)	a	327)	a		
280)	d	304)	c	328)	b		

Answers with comments

1)   b   The dose rate is 2 mg/kg.
Therefore a 15 kg dog requires $2 \ mg \times 15 \ = 30 \ mg$.
The drug is in a 50 mg/ml solution.
As the dog requires 30 mg, it will need
$\frac{30}{50} ml = \frac{3}{5} ml = 0.6 \ ml$.

2)   b   If you have difficulty remembering this, try thinking of
the label on the thiopentone bottle: a 100 ml bottle of
2.5% thiopentone contains 2.5 g.

3)   d   The total dose required per 24 hours will be
$30 \times 25 \ mg = 750 \ mg$.
Therefore each injection must contain 250 mg.
A 5% solution contains 50 mg/ml
So $\frac{250}{50} ml = 5 \ ml$ must be given at each injection.

4)   b   If the dose rate is 25 mg/kg, then a 40 kg dog requires
$40 \times 25 \ mg = 1000 \ mg$ each day.
If the dose is to be split, then each injection must
contain 500 mg.
If the suspension contains 150 mg/ml, then each
injection must be
$\frac{500}{150} = 3.3 \ ml$.

5)   b   If the dose is 50 mg/kg/24 hours, the total daily dose for
a 4 kg cat will be $4 \times 50 = 200 \ mg$.
Therefore each daily dose must contain 100 mg.
So the cat will need 1 tablet twice daily for 10 days
= 20 tablets.

6)   c

7)   d   However carefully it is done, the introduction of a catheter may introduce infection or cause damage to the urethral or bladder wall that may predispose to opportunist infection.

8)   b   If the dose is 10 mg/kg, then the dose for an 18 kg dog is $18 \times 10 = 180\ mg$.
A 7.5% solution contains 75 mg/ml.
The correct volume for the dog is therefore
$\frac{180}{75} = 2.4\ ml$.

9)   a   A 2.5% solution contains 2.5 g in 100 ml. Therefore 50 ml of the same solution will contain 1.25 g.

10) b   If the dose rate is 50 mg/kg, then the dose for a 20 kg dog will be $50 \times 20 = 1000\ mg$. A 10% solution contains 100 mg/ml. Therefore this dog requires $\frac{1000}{100} = 10\ ml$ of the solution.

11) c

12) b

13) c   But it does sometimes require sedation.

14) d   Other common signs of pain are tachycardia, pale mucous membranes and pupillary dilation.

15) a   Only the use of a gastrostomy tube carries with it the risk of peritonitis, because only in this case is a laparotomy required to insert it — i.e. an incision into the peritoneal cavity.

16) b   Anything that might cause excessive straining, or very firm faeces, would not be used following anal sac surgery.

17) c   Ill and recumbent animals require fewer calories, as they are expending less on movement — but must have enough to produce sufficient heat to keep warm. They may require increased protein for tissue repair.

18) d   Research in human hospital patients shows that people tend to make a more rapid recovery if they have a nice view from their bed and are given plenty of cheerful attention!

19)   c   Saline solution may be dangerous in a young animal as the electrolytes can be absorbed in the colon, and disrupt the electrolyte balance of the body.

20)   b

21)   b

22)   d

23)   c   Maintenance requirements are calculated at 40 ml/kg/24 hours. This is made up of 20 ml/kg urinary loss and 20 ml/kg insensible loss (from the skin and respiratory tract). The maintenance requirement of a 10 kg dog will be $40 \times 10 = 400 \; ml/24 \; hours$, so 1.5 times maintenance will be $1.5 \times 400 = 600 \; ml/24 \; hours$. For the second part of the question, you start by saying *600 ml to be given in 24 hours*. So in 1 hr, $\frac{600}{24} = 25 \; ml$ will be needed. You can then work out how much should be given per minute, which is $\frac{25}{60} \; ml = 0.42 \; ml$. This is just under half a ml. And if the drip set delivers 15 drops per ml, then 0.42 ml will be just under half, which will be about 6 drops per minute.

24)   b

25)   d   The normal Central Venous Pressure is between 3 and 7 cm water. 2 cm is therefore low, and so more fluids should be given. A dog in danger of overhydration would have a CVP *above* the normal range.

26)   b   This question is best divided into two parts. First, work out how much dextrose is required to make 500 ml of a 2.5% solution.
We know that 100 ml of a 2.5% solution contains 2.5 g.
So 500 ml of a 2.5% solution will contain 12.5 g.
Now work out how much of a 50% dextrose solution will contain 12.5 g of dextrose.
500 ml of a 50% dextrose solution will contain 250 g.
We only want 12.5 g. So we will need
$\frac{12.5}{250} \times 500 \; ml = 25 \; ml$.

27)   c

28)   a   Plasma starts to deteriorate very fast in store unless it is frozen.

29) c

30) a   Any longer than this and a thick fibrin sheath will form round the catheter, which is then released into the circulation when the catheter is removed.

31) d   Sometimes just either 7.35 or 7.4 is given as an answer to this question. 7.4 is a reasonable approximation, but 7.35 is more accurate.

32) c

33) a   Make sure that you can name a use for the other three anticoagulants.

34) d   Alkalosis is caused by a lack of or decrease in acid — i.e. in the hydrogen ion concentration. The usual way that a body loses hydrogen ions is by vomiting, which leads to a loss of hydrochloric acid from the stomach.

35) c   All the rest are colloids.

36) a   This is the only common intravenous fluid that is hypertonic. Administration of a hypertonic solution on its own may lead to dehydration of the interstitial fluid (and possibly the ICF) — so great care must be taken. Its main use is in the treatment of circulatory collapse.

37) c   And sodium is the main cation in extracellular fluid.

38) c   Losses through the skin (sweat and lacrimal glands) are often included with inevitable loss.

39) d   These are the main ions throughout the extracellular fluid. They are the main constituents of most crystalloid intravenous fluids.

40) c   A burette allows a measured volume to run through into it from the bag of intravenous fluids — say 150 ml. This amount can then be given, without any danger of the rest of the bag running through as well.

41) b   Hartmann's solution is the most suitable because it is purely an electrolyte solution, and does not contain any dextrose.

42) b   Hartmann's solution is the most suitable for the replacement of both water and electrolytes, such as occurs in diarrhoea.

43)   b   PCV can certainly be used to estimate fluid loss, as in a given animal it tends to rise by about 1% for each 10 ml/kg fluid loss. However, this can only be an estimate, as it is rare that the normal PCV of the animal is known.

44)   b   Intra-osseous needle placement should only be done following a strict aseptic regime, because of the risk of bone infection.

45)   a   Any of the other three signs may occur quite rapidly either during or shortly after a blood transfusion.

46)   b   Anaemia, over-hydration and renal failure will all result in a decrease in serum protein.

47)   a   For longer term storage, serum should be frozen.

48)   a   They are usually seen when immature erythrocytes are released into the circulation following a loss of circulating erythrocytes — for example after a road traffic accident or a haemolytic episode. Reticulocytes might be seen in the same situation.

49)   a   Make sure you can give an example of the use of heparin, sodium nitrate and sodium fluoride as anticoagulants.

50)   b

51)   a

52)   d   A low PCV and low rbc suggests a recent loss of red blood cells. The relatively high reticulocyte count suggests that the bone marrow is working overtime to replenish the deficit by releasing immature red blood cells into the circulation. Reticulocytes are red blood cells showing nuclear remnants in the form of a network of threads in the cytoplasm. In bone marrow hypoplasia, chronic renal disease and in FeLV, the bone marrow activity is depressed, and large numbers of reticulocytes are not likely to be seen.

53)   c

54)   a

55)   b

56)   d

57) b Rouleaux is most common where there is an increase in fibrinogen or globulin in the blood (except in horses, where it is seen in normal blood).

58) b

59) b

60) d

61) d

62) a

63) c Neutropaenia is, of course, a LACK of neutrophils. Large numbers of neutrophils — a neutrophilia — might well be seen in infectious inflammatory conditions.

64) c Creatinine kinase (an enzyme) increases in the presence of severe muscle damage.

65) d

66) d

67) c

68) c A coenurus contains many scolices, a cysticercoid contains a single evaginated scolex (not invaginated), and a hydatid contains many scolices loose within the fluid of the cyst.

69) a *Aelurostrongylus* is the cat lungworm. The eggs are coughed up and swallowed, and so appear in the faeces of the cat.

70) b Except for the insect growth regulators, such as are found in *Program*, all insecticides have, potentially, some effect of the CNS.

71) d *Dipylidium caninum* is the commonest tapeworm of the dog and cat that has the flea or louse as its intermediate host. It doesn't usually cause disease in the final host.

72) a *Trichuris vulpis* is the whipworm, *Toxocara* is a roundworm, and *Uncinaria stenocephala* a hookworm.

73) b It takes until about three weeks of age for larvae entering the pup through the placenta or by ingestion through the milk to mature into adult worms in the intestine.

74) d

75) a

76) a

Warning: illegal if copied

77) c *Aracheopsyllus* is the hedgehog flea, and *Pulex irritans* is the human flea!

78) b

79) d The mature tapeworm tends only to be seen in areas where dogs can scavenge the carcases of dead sheep.

80) b This tapeworm is usually found in dogs, but may occur in cats as well.

81) b

82) c This fact is important when advising clients on worming a bitch during pregnancy.

83) b

84) a

85) c

86) d *T. taeniaeformis* has rodents such as mice and rats as its intermediate host.

87) c

88) d Fenbendazole is effective against nematodes and cestodes, and niclosamide and praziquantel only against cestodes.

89) d

90) c In this, *T. cati* differs from *T. canis*, which is able to cause intra-uterine infection.

91) b *Cnemidocoptes* lives in tunnels in proliferated epidermis. All the others are visible either to the naked eye or with a hand lens.

92) c *Toxoplasma gondii* is a ubiquitous organism, present throughout the environment. Cats may be tested negative for *T. gondii* antibodies, only to get infected the day after testing, whereas wearing rubber goves while gardening will protect against infection from the soil.

93) c

94) a

95) b Because it is a tapeworm, not an ectoparasite.

96) b But you might hear it mentioned — it is the dog heartworm, which must be considered in routine worming programmes in most parts or the United States of America and elsewhere.

97)   b   And is said to cause *follicular mange.*

98)   a   The final host is the animal that hosts the adult, sexually-reproducing stage of the parasite — i.e. in this case the adult tapeworm. The hydatid cyst is an intermediate (juvenile) form.

99)   b   Even in ideal warm, moist conditions, a fertile *Toxocara* egg takes 10 days to 3 weeks to develop to the infective stage. So contamination with really fresh dog faeces is less of a worry than contact with areas where they have been until washed away by the rain, leaving infective larvae behind...

100)   d   It is not red meat *per se*, but almost *any* meat that might be infected and pregnant women are advised not to eat any undercooked meat (as often seen at barbeques in summer) as this might be a source of *T. gondii*.

101)   c   They may become infective in under a week.

102)   b   Cat lungworm is probably underdiagnosed in the U.K., as many cats probably harbour the worm, but only those with quite a heavy burden will show clinical signs such as coughing.

103)   c   Grisovin is only used parenterally. Take note, though, of the alternative answers, especially b and d. The fact that it is teratogenic means that it should only be handled with gloves on, and the likelihood of *enteric disturbances* means that clients should be warned!

104)   a   This parasite rarely causes clinical signs in the final host. It is commonest where dogs are able to scavenge sheep carcases.The second sub-species affects horses, with hounds that are fed on horse meat being the final host.

105)   b   *Trombicula autumnalis* only affects its host in the late summer and autumn. All the rest are true!

106)   d

107)   b   The presence of a grass run which cannot be satisfactorily disinfected means that eggs passed in the faeces can develop on the grass to the infective larval stage.

108)   c

109) b   Neither a nor c are true — but the fact that there is a risk of human infection, which may be serious or fatal, must be communicated to the owner, and will often influence the choice as to whether or not the dog is to be treated.

110) c

111) c

112) b   When canine parvovirus first arrived in the U.K., FIE vaccines were given to dogs to try to produce some degree of immunity to the virus.

113) b

114) b   Cats suffering from chlamydiosis are often quite healthy, apart from a purulent conjunctivitis.

115) d

116) b

117) a

118) d

119) a

120) c   *Bordatella* causes kennel cough (infectious tracheo-bronchitis), canine adenovirus causes respiratory disease or infectious canine hepatitis, and canine parainfluenza virus causes respiratory disease, and is the *Pi* element in many dog vaccines.

121) b

122) c   Maternal antibodies to canine distemper are usually lost between six and nine weeks of age. Vaccination after this time will produce immunity in over 95% of vaccinated dogs, but dogs that are not vaccinated have to rely on meeting small doses of *field virus* to stimulate the development of immunity, and this takes some time to happen.

123) d   Urban areas where there are large numbers of unvaccinated dogs are the main reservoirs of distemper virus in the U.K.

124) c   Vaccination of wild foxes against rabies using an oral vaccine in bait has been the single most effective measure in halting the spread of rabies on the European mainland.

125) d

126) d

127) c

128) c

129) d   The presence of tongue ulcers is the most obvious sign that differentiates FRTV and FCV infection.

130) c

131) a   Classically, the signs of canine distemper are: cough, pyrexia, green oculo-nasal discharge, hyperkeratosis of pads, and nervous signs. A dog exhibiting several of these signs together is likely to be suffering from canine distemper.

132) d   *Spilopsyllus cuniculi* is the rabbit flea, which acts as a vector for the myxomatosis virus.

133) a   An adjuvant, is a substance added to an inactivated vaccine to increase its antigenic effect. Aluminium hydroxide and mineral oil are the two usual examples.

134) a   **b** is wrong because a lot of dogs contract distemper as a sub-clinical or mild disease; **c** is wrong because the disease can last for six to eight weeks, and **d** is incorrect because many of the old dogs that show chorea (nervous signs due to the distemper virus) have had the virus in the body since early middle age.

135) a   The disease is seen much more commonly in males than females. They tend to contract the disease via bite wounds.

136) b   The toxoid stimulates the production of antibodies, whereas an antitoxin provides antibodies to the toxin. The antitoxin is given when there is an immediate danger of infection in an unvaccinated animal — most commonly in veterinary practice in horses, for protection against tetanus.

137) b   Rabies can affect any mammal, but does not affect birds.

138)   c   Remember that canine adenovirus 1 produces the disease infectious canine hepatitis. Infection with canine adenovirus-2 produces respiratory disease. However, vaccination using a live vaccine derived from CAV-2 protects against both diseases without the side effects (e.g. corneal oedema) produced by the CAV-1 live vaccine.

139)   c

140)   b   Corneal oedema may occur after vaccination, or associated with the disease.

141)   b   *L. icterohaemorrhagiae* primarily affects the liver, causing the jaundice suggested by its name (icterus = jaundice).

142)   a   The persistence of the right aortic arch instead of the left leaves the oesophagus caught in a loop of blood vessels. This usually only becomes apparent after weaning, when the inability to take in solid food leads to persistent vomiting. If either or both of the ductus arteriosus or foramen ovale persist after birth, it results in mixing of blood from left and right sides ofthe heart, and less efficient oxygenation — it does not interfere with the intake of food.

143)   b

144)   d

145)   d   If the diarrhoea had originated in the large intestine, any blood released would be seen in the faeces as fresh blood, rather than the changed, partly digested blood that is seen in melaena. Blood produced in the small intestine is acted on by the digestive enzymes — there are no digestive enzymes produced in the large intestine.

146)   a   Constant muscle activity may lead to hyperthermia.

147)   c

148)   d   Atopic dermatitis is caused by inhaled allergens.

149)   b   Waste nitrogen in monitored in the circulation of the mammal as urea and creatinine.

150)   b

151)   d   Raw egg white contains avidin, which binds to biotin and makes it unavailable to the animal.

152) a   The signs of Cushing's disease are similar to those that may be seen in long-term corticosteroid therapy.

153) b   Vasopressin is also known as anti-diuretic hormone. It is secreted by the posterior pituitary gland, and controls the re-absorption of water in the distal convoluted tubule of the kidney.

154) c   Endocardiosis is the condition where *cauliflower like growths* develop on the valves of the heart. It is commonly seen in small breeds such as King Charles spaniels and in poodles.

155) a   Vitamin A is stored in the liver, and toxicity can occur if liver makes up too high a proportion of the diet.

156) c

157) b   In malabsorption syndrome, nutrients are not taken from the lumen of the gut into the circulation. Both stress (with increased secretion of adrenomedullary hormones and glucocorticoids) and the sudden overconsumption of short chain carbohydrates can cause the blood glucose level to exceed the renal threshhold — glucose will then appear in the urine.

158) c   Prehepatic jaundice occurs before the blood reaches the liver — i.e. there is excessive breakdown of red blood cells in the circulation. In posthepatic jaundice the liver cannot get rid of the breakdown products of red cell destruction in the normal way (in the bile) — for example because of bile duct obstruction.

159) d   Ketones are a product of fat breakdown.

160) a

161) d

162) b

163) b

164) a   Acute, as opposed to chronic, renal failure in the dog or cat is commonly oliguric or even anuric.

165) d   In nephrotic syndrome, there is protein loss in the urine. This results in a lowering of the amount of plasma protein, and a decrease in the osmotic pressure of plasma — hence the ascites and oedema.

166) d

167) a

168) b   Otherwise known as Addison's disease — this condition has no effect on the skin. Hyperadrenocorticalism is Cushing's disease.

169) a

170) b   Unless the cat was also suffering from renal failure! A low magnesium diet, antibiotics and urinary acidifiers may all be employed in the treatment of FUS.

171) c   Pulmonary oedema is not usually seen in right sided heart failure, as inefficient pumping of blood on the right side of the heart leads to back flow into the systemic (not the pulmonary) circulation. So ascites, a jugular pulse and spenomegaly may all be seen.

172) c   It is not characterised by pulmonary oedema, but by the presence of a space occupying lesion in the thorax. Why this gives rise to periosteal bone formation in the distal limbs is not known.

173) d   Struvite is otherwise known as triple phosphate, or magnesium ammonium phosphate. It is the commonest type of crystal seen in dogs and cats.

174) a   A rise in ALT indicates hepatocellular damage. Bilirubin is indicative of bile duct obstruction, creatinine of renal insufficiency, and a high lipase is commonly seen in cases of pancreatitis.

175) d   See above!

176) d   A water deprivation test is commonly used to investigate a possible case of diabetes insipidus.

177) d

178) a

179) b   Most cats that have made the mistake of playing with a toad and getting a mouthful of toad venom — which is unpleasant but not dangerous — never do it again, and frogs are usually safe from that cat as well!

180) a   Calcium edetate is used in lead poisoning, ethanol in ethylene glycol (antifreeze) poisoning, and vitamin K in coumarin rodent bait poisoning.

89

181) d

182) d

183) b Lindane is an organo chlorine — rarely now seen. Can you remember the names of products that contain Dichlovos, Fenthion and Malathion?

184) c

185) b

186) b Dogs suffering from ethylene glycol poisoning develop pulmonary congestion and renal failure.

187) a Engine coolant is a source of ethylene glycol.

188) d

189) a

190) a

191) c Cholecalciferol was introduced as a rodenticide claimed to be less toxic to non-target species than the coumarin rodenticides. It causes hypercalcaemia, which results in renal failure, hypertension and heart irregularities.

192) d It is very rare indeed that any attempt to prevent death after ingestion of paraquat is successful.

193) b Just because human beings can eat large quantities of chocolate without obvious toxic effects, many owners do not realise that relatively small quantities of chocolate can be fatal to a dog. (It is thought that 10 g per kg may cause signs, and 100 g per kg bodyweight may cause death.)

194) a

195) d The film/focal distance is a red herring — multiply the exposure without a grid by the grid factor.

196) a

197) a

198) a

199) d The filament and the target are both made of tungsten.

200) a

201) d

202) a

203) b Or to be more accurate, on the pubic symphysis between the acetabula.

204) b
205) c
206) c
207) a
208) b
209) b
210) b Note that the question concerns the primary beam, not the scattered radiation.
211) c
212) a Exposures of the abdomen are usually taken on expiration, so the diaphragm is as far forward as possible, and the abdomen is as thin as posible.
213) a A lead-lined apron will protect against scattered radiation but will not give sufficient protection against the primary beam.
214) d
215) a
216) b Photographers sometimes just refer to it as *thio*.
217) d
218) d This type of abscess is often seen in reptiles. Surgical excision of the whole abscess is the only treatment.
219) d
220) a
221) d Often described as a *wart*.
222) b A plaster should, in general, enclose the joint above and the joint below the fracture line to provide immobilisation.
223) a A sutured operative wound in correctly prepared skin is a clean wound. The oral mucosa cannot be made aseptic, so the wound is described as *clean-contaminated*.
224) c Mucus accumulates very rapidly round a foreign body in the respiratory tract. If the tube is not cleaned regularly, it can become obstructed.
225) d Extension splints are most often used to stabilise fractures in the proximal limb, where the fracture is surrounded by a large mass of muscle, and so cannot be stabilised with a plaster cast.

226) a Whereas a xenograft comes from a different species.
227) c In cats, following bite wounds, cellulitis often precedes the formation of an abscess.
228) b
229) d
230) a
231) b Any word ending in *-otomy* means to make a temporary opening in the wall of a viscus.
232) c In fracture disease, rigidity of the joints also leads to muscle atrophy.
233) c
234) d If the situation is that desperate, and the patient is cyanotic, you don't waste time on skin preparation!
235) a A dry dressing will not encourage sloughing — the black necrotic tissue will remain covering the wound. Wet dressings — particularly alginate or hydrocolloid dressings — keep the necrotic tissue moist and encourage it to slough.
236) b The term *organisation* is only used when the end result of the healing process is scar tissue. When the tissue returns to normal it is termed repair or resolution.
237) d
238) d
239) c Calculus and tartar are both terms for the hard mineral deposit that forms on teeth.
240) b
241) a
242) d
243) b
244) b
245) b
246) c The presence of a drain will have no effect on the healing of the original wound, as drains are usually placed through an incision separate to the surgical wound.
247) a
248) a

249) b By the post-operative period, hypothermia may have developed already! However, fluids will, of course, aid a rapid recovery, and replace any fluid deficit through haemorrhage or reduced intake in the peri-operative period.

250) b A hypothermic animal usually has a decreased heart rate.

251) a

252) b There is also a small amount (about 5%) sodium hydroxide.

253) b There are various methods for working out flow rates. Minute volume is about 200 ml/kg/minute (less in large and more in smaller animals). A Magill circuit only requires a flow rate of about 1 × minute volume. So in this case, minute volume $= 200 \times 30 = 6000 \; ml/min = 6 \, l/min$.

254) d

255) b

256) a A modified Bain is used more frequently in veterinary practice than a standard Bain.

257) c

258) a

259) a A Lack circuit should be used with a flow rate of approximately 1 × MV. Assuming a minute volume of approximately 200 ml/kg/min, a 15 kg dog will require a flow rate of $15 \times 200 \; ml = 3000 \; ml = 3 \, litres$ total gas flow rate.

260) b A Magill circuit requires a flow rate of approximately 1 × MV. Assuming a minute volume of approximately 200 ml/kg/min, a 25 kg dog will have a minute volume of $200 \times 25 = 5000 \; ml = 5 \, litres$ total gas flow rate.

261) b An Ayre's T-piece requires a flow rate of approximately 2.5 × MV. Assuming a minute volume of approximately 200 ml/kg/min, an 8 kg dog will have a minute volume of $200 \times 8 = 1600 \; ml = 1.6 \, litres$. Since the Ayre's T-piece requires a flow rate of 2.5 × MV, the total gas flow rate required will be $2.5 \times 1.6 = 4 \, litres$.

262) b If the dose rate is 3 mg/kg, a 6 kg cat will require $6 \times 3 = 18\ mg$. If there are 12 mg/ml of solution, this cat will require 1.5 ml.

263) b 1.25% thiopentone contains 12.5 mg/ml. A 3.75 kg cat requires $3.75 \times 10\ mg = 37.5\ mg$. If there are 12.5 mg/ml, then the volume required to anaesthetise the cat will be $\frac{37.5}{12.5}ml = 3\ ml$.

264) a 2.5% thiopentone contains 25 mg/ml. A 25 kg labrador requires $25 \times 10\ mg = 250\ mg$. If there are 25 mg/ml, then the volume required to anaesthetise the cat will be $\frac{250}{25}ml = 10\ ml$.

265) c Remember that the central venous pressure is measured via a catheter placed in the first instance in a jugular vein, and passed down towards the heart. The first chamber it reaches will be the right atrium.

266) d With any of the other regimes, there will not be enough cardiac compressions to carry oxygenated blood around the body.

267) d

268) d Or 5 g.

269) c

270) b

271) d

272) a

273) a

274) b

275) b

276) d

277) a

278) b

279) b In nearly all questions about emergency resuscitation, the answer is *establish an airway*!

280) d

281) d

282) b An anaesthetic agent with a high therapeutic index may sometimes be used in total intravenous anaesthesia — e.g. Saffan.

283)   d   This is the correct answer! It requires a little anticipation and careful observation not to remove it too early.

284)   c   A closed to-and-fro circuit should not be used with nitrous oxide as it is very difficult to predict when to refill the bag with nitrous oxide present — with a resultant risk of the patient becoming hypoxic.

285)   a

286)   c

287)   d

288)   a

289)   a

290)   b

291)   d

292)   a

293)   d

294)   c

295)   b

296)   a

297)   c   Boyle's bottle can be used with a mixture of gases, but the other statements are all true. Because the bottle is not insulated, the liquid inside will cool during administration (unless it's a very hot day), so during the course of administration, the amount that vapourises will decrease.

298)   c   When used on its own, ketamine produces an increase in muscle tone.

299)   b

300)   a   Respiratory depression is greater than with thiopentone.

301)   b

302)   c

303)   a   Tachycardia is often a response to pain.

304)   c   Cardiac and respiratory depression is often marked with neuroleptanalgesia.

305)   c

306)   a   But this faster respiration is often very shallow.

307)   d   A Bain circuit requires a flow rate of approximately $2.5 \times$ MV. Assuming a minute volume of 200 ml/kg/minute, then a 20 kg dog has a minute volume of $200 \times 20 = 4000\ ml = 4\ l$. The total gas flow should therefore be $2.5 \times 4 = 10\ l/min$.

308)   d

309)   b

310)   c   A 2.5% solution contains 25 mg/ml. If the dose rate is 10 mg/kg, then a 35 kg labrador will require $35 \times 10\ mg = 350\ mg$. If there are 25 mg in 1 ml, then the volume needed will be $\frac{350}{25}\ ml = 14\ ml$.

311)   d

312)   c

313)   d

314)   d

315)   b

316)   d

317)   d

318)   b

319)   a

320)   a

321)   a

322)   b

323)   a

324)   a

325)   c

326)   b

327)   a   It is important NOT to screw the stopper down tight, as otherwise, pressure will build up as the liquid gradually evaporates.

328)   b   All this will do is to stir up any dust and get it flying round the room.

329)   b   Because it is non-irritant to mucosae.

330)   d

331)   c

332) d   In other words, any of the other possible answers will reduce the efficiency of autoclaving — poor cleaning or overloading the autoclave.

333) d   All the others require a size 3 or 5.

334) d

335) d

336) c   A diet for a heavily pregnant bitch will include fat as an energy source, but not be too high in fibre, as she has little enough room in her abdomen for food, without fibre filling the gut.

337) b   First stage labour is the dilation of the cervix, and third stage labour is the delivery of the afterbirth. Second stage labour is defined as the stage of delivery of the young, and dystocia is a difficulty with birth.

338) c   This is the membrane that forms the *water-bag* that ruptures before the first fetus can be born. Pups may be born still largely enclosed within the *slime bag* or amnion.

339) b   It is not until after 42 days of pregnancy that encysted *Toxocara canis* larvae start to migrate to the gut and the puppies in the uterus.

340) b

341) d

342) a   They are hypothermic compared to the adult dog.

343) c

344) d

345) d

346) a

347) a   Remember that in the bitch the discharge is green, but in the queen it is brown.

348) a   A drop in body temperature of up to 1 deg C (2 deg F) is common shortly before the onset of parturition.

349) b

350) c   An induced ovulator is a species where the female remains almost constantly *in season* unless mated. The act of mating stimulates the release of the ova from the ovary.